Recent Advances in

Dermatology 1

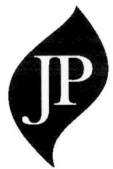

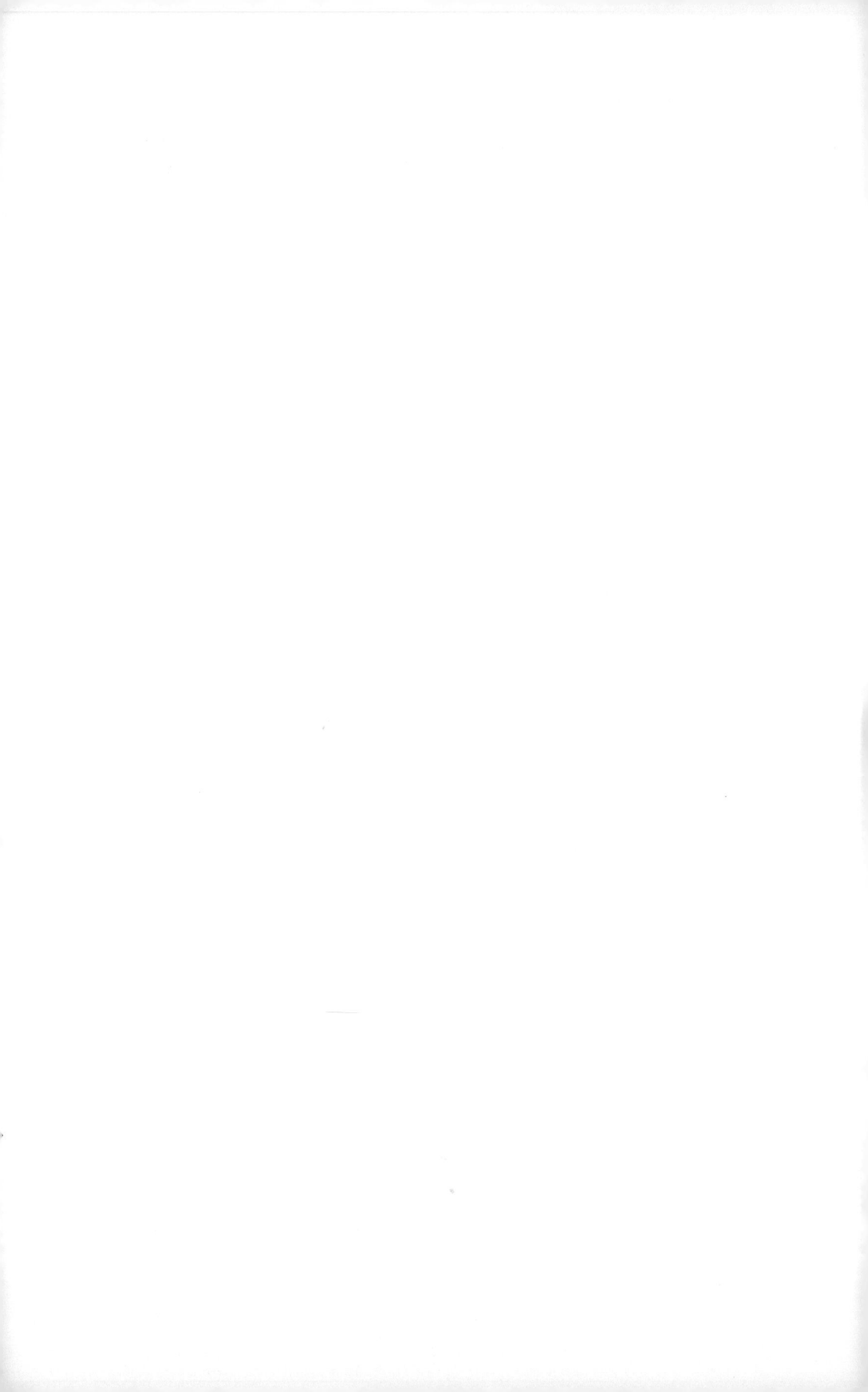

Recent Advances in

Dermatology 1

Shirin Zaheri BSc (Hons) MBBS MRCP PGCME
Consultant Dermatologist & Senior Honorary Lecturer
Charing Cross Hospital
Imperial College Healthcare NHS Trust
London, UK

Iaisha Ali MB ChB MRCP MSc
Consultant Dermatologist
HCA Harley Street Clinic
London, UK

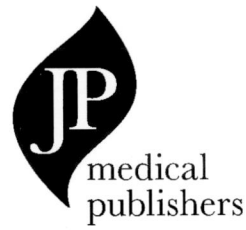

JP
medical
publishers

London • Panama City • New Delhi

© 2019 JP Medical Ltd.
Published by JP Medical Ltd,
83 Victoria Street, London, SW1H 0HW, UK
Tel: +44 (0)20 3170 8910
Fax: +44 (0)20 3008 6180
Email: info@jpmedpub.com
Web: www.jpmedpub.com

ISBN: 978-1-909836-58-7

British Library Cataloguing in Publication Data
A catalogue record for this book is available from the British Library

Library of Congress Cataloging in Publication Data
A catalog record for this book is available from the Library of Congress

Preface

For over 50 years the *Recent Advances* series has provided timely reviews on topics of current interest across a number of medical specialties. This is the first title in the series to cover dermatology. Our specialty has witnessed enormous changes in the last few years and made quantum leaps in terms of new treatments, especially with the advent of biologics. Evidence generated from high quality research has underpinned major changes in clinical practice and accentuated the need for up-to-date information sources.

This volume has been written to reflect these changes and highlights key advances in the management of eczema, genital dermatology and urticara, to name a few. It is not intended to be an exhaustive textbook, but a primer which provides up-to-date, evidence-based information and guidance for clinicians involved in the care of patients with dermatological conditions. We have written this book primarily as an update for trainees wishing to keep abreast of important advances prior to membership and fellowship exams. The chapters, distilled from existing published research, have been written by well-established clinicians in their field of expertise. We hope you find this first volume in the *Recent Advances in Dermatology series* a useful resource for learning and clinical practice.

Shirin Zaheri
Iaisha Ali
October 2018

Contents

Acknowledgements

The editors and publishers are very grateful to all the authors for their hard work. We thank our families, friends and colleagues for their invaluable support and patience during the writing of this book.

Shirin Zaheri
Iaisha Ali

Dedication

I would like to dedicate this book to my beloved brother in law, Mahmoud Honardoost (1960-2007). He always told me 'the world is your oyster' and you could achieve anything if you set your mind to it.

Shirin Zaheri

I would like to dedicate this book to my patients who have made my work as a dermatologist worthwhile. I learn something new every day

Iaisha Ali

Chapter 1

Oral lichen planus: aetiopathogenesis, clinical presentation and management

Manpreet K Lakhan, Jane Setterfield

INTRODUCTION

Lichen planus (LP) is a chronic T-cell mediated autoimmune disorder with a wide spectrum of clinical presentation and severity of disease. It may be localised to one site, e.g. scalp, nails, oral mucosa, or, it may become a more widespread mucocutaneous inflammatory condition affecting multiple sites, including the skin, oral cavity, anogenital skin, external ear, conjunctiva, lachrymal ducts, and oesophagus. Importantly it can result in significant scarring and stricture formation. The incidence of this more severe form varies between 0.22% and 1% of the adult population worldwide [1]. In contrast, oral lichen planus (OLP) seems to be more frequent with a reported incidence between 0.5% and 2.2% of the population being rare in children but presenting more usually in adults during their fourth to sixth decades with a female predominance of 2:1 [1]. The commonest oral lesions are reticular striae, but several clinical subtypes are recognised. Oral lesions may be long-lasting with a potential lifetime risk for malignant transformation in approximately 1% patients [3]. Dermatologists and other clinicians examining these patients must be aware of this risk and refer promptly when lesions are failing to resolve with treatment or are atypical.

AETIOPATHOGENESIS

The pathogenesis of LP is not yet fully understood but many factors have been implicated including genetic association, immune dysregulation, infections, drugs and contact factors among others.

Genetics

The major histocompatibility complex (MHC) region on chromosome 6 has been implicated in many autoimmune disorders. In a phenome-wide association study

Manpreet K Lakhan MBChB, MRCP 1 St John's Institute of Dermatology, Guy's & St Thomas' Hospitals NHS Foundation Trust, UK.

Jane Setterfield BDS, MBBS, MD, FRCP 1, 2 Department of Oral Medicine, Guy's Hospital Dental Institute, King's College London, UK, Email: jane.setterfield@kcl.ac.uk (for correspondence).

(PheWAS) of 7481 subjects from the Marshfield Clinic Personalised Medicine Research Project in Wisconsin, USA where disease phenotypes (defined by their ICD9 codes) were mapped to this region, LP was the most significant phenotype association [4]. Haplotype HLA DBQ1*05:01 had the strongest link with LP. The study further demonstrated an association between a single peptide nucleotide (SNP) rs1794275 together with 5 other SNPs across the MHC. These are also associated with multiple sclerosis and type 1 diabetes. In a similarly well defined sub-group of scarring LP, the vulvovaginal gingival syndrome LP (VVG-LP), a strong association was reported with the DQB1*0201 allele. The authors have shown 28/35 (80%) patients having the DQB1*0201 allele versus 74/177 (41.8%) of healthy control subjects [5]. No other subgroups of LP were associated with this allele.

Other possible associations

Hepatitis C: There is evidence in the literature to suggest that in some geographic regions, OLP is associated with hepatitis C virus (HCV) infection. The association is stronger in Japanese and Mediteranean populations where the prevalence of hepatitis C is greater. The association may be related to their predisposition to other extrahepatic complications of HCV infection such as cryoglobulinaemia. Northern European patients are rarely associated with HCV [6].

Drugs: A wide range of drugs have been linked with lichenoid rashes. These include antimicrobials, antihypertensives, antimalarials, antidepressants, anticonvulsants, diuretics, metals, non-steroidal anti-inflammatory drugs (NSAIDs) and more recently intravenous immunoglobulins [2].

Anxiety/depression/stress: Patients with LP, in particular erosive LP have a higher reported incidence of anxiety and depression. Although exacerbations of OLP may be associated with episodes of anxiety and stress, a cause-and-effect relationship has not been identified [6].

Autoimmunity: There is an increased frequency of other autoimmune diseases in patients with OLP. A Taiwanese study of 12,427 LP patients and 49,708 age- and gender-matched controls drawn from a National database reported significant associations among LP patients with systemic lupus erythematosus, Sjögren's syndrome, dermatomyositis, vitiligo and alopecia areata [7]. In a Swedish study, data from 956 patients with OLP and 1029 controls were collected using a standardized registration method. Patients with OLP used thyroid preparations ($p < 0.001$) and NSAIDs ($p < 0.01$) in higher proportions compared to controls. A multivariate logistic regression model demonstrated that levothyroxine was associated with OLP and by implication hypothyroidism [8]. In a subgroup of VVG-LP patients, 12/40 (30%) had another autoimmune disease with thyroid disorders present in six [5].

Immune dysregulation: LP is a T-cell mediated autoimmune disease. Histologically, it is characterised by a dense band of lymphocytes just below the epithelial basement membrane zone associated with saw-toothed rete ridges and apoptotic keratinocytes. Direct immunofluorescence (DIF) shows a ragged fibrin band (**Figure 1.1**).

Evidence from chronic graft versus host disease suggests that lymphocytes are targeting antigens on keratinocytes that they recognise as foreign giving rise to lesions indistinguishable clinically and histologically from OLP [9]. Antigens may include altered self or extrinsic antigens (e.g. food, drugs, bacteria, viruses, dental materials). The

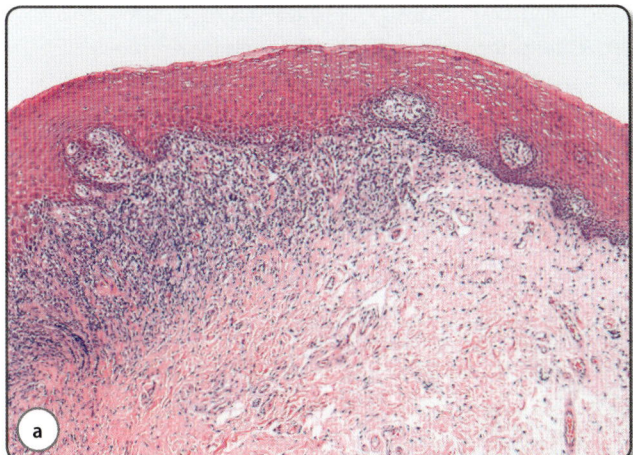

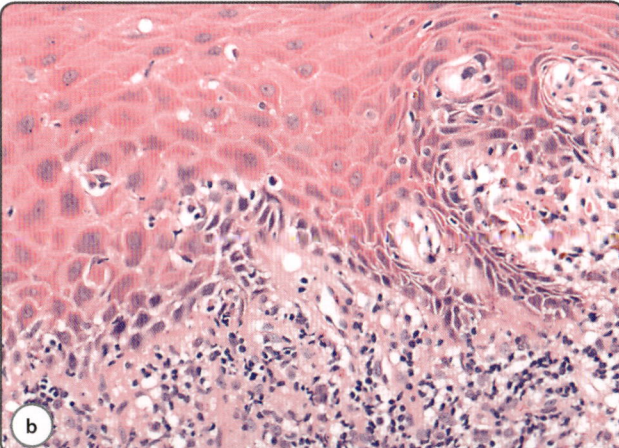

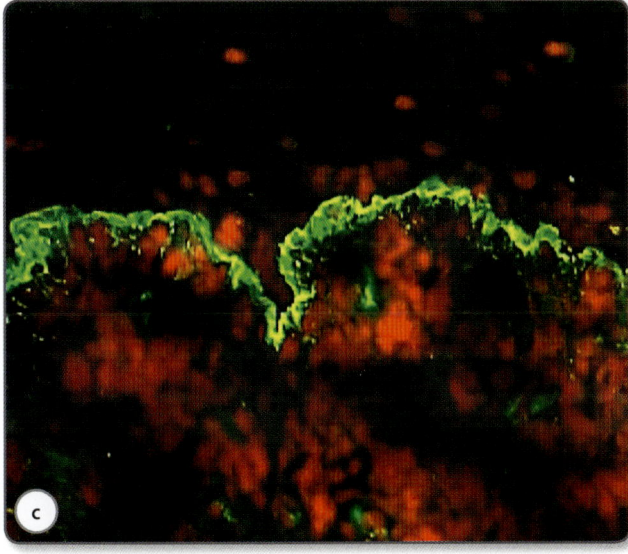

Figure 1.1 (a) Low-power view showing a sub-epithelial lymphocytic infiltrate that is well demarcated laterally. There is a mild degree of basal cell loss and some reactive rete hyperplasia focally. (Courtesy of Edward Odell, Oral Pathology, King's College London, London). (b) At higher power lymphocytes are seen associated with apoptosis in the basal and supra basal layers with basement membrane thickening, basal squamoid change and melanin dropout (Courtesy of Edward Odell, Oral Pathology, King's College London, London). (c) Ragged fibrin band characteristically seen in lichen planus with absence of a homogenous band of immunoglobulins or complement (Courtesy of Balbir Bhogal, St John's Institute of Dermatology, King's College London, London).

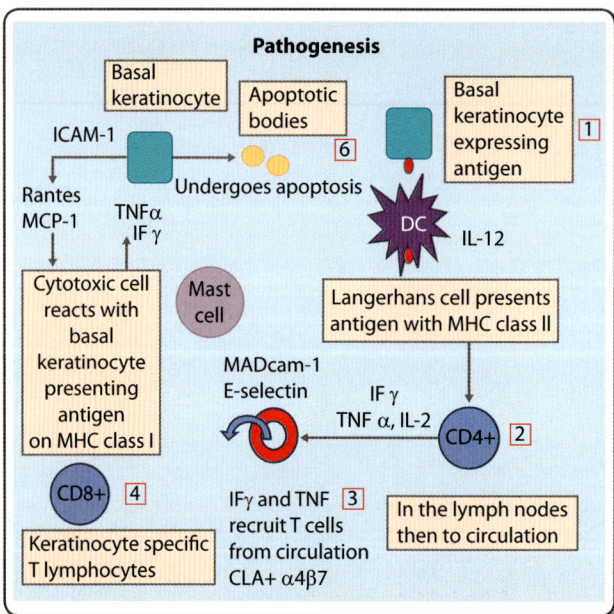

Figure 1.2 Potential pathogenic mechanisms for OLP. 1. Langerhans cells take up antigen and are induced by TNF and/or local inflammatory mediators to migrate to the local lymph node (LN). 2. From the local LN, CD4+ T cells preferentially move to the oral mucosa. 3. TNF-α, IF-γ and other cytoines induce E-selectin and MADcam-1 on surface of blood vessels. This leads to the selective recruitment of activated skin homing (CLA+) and gut α4β7 homing lymphocytes from the circulation. VCAM-1 is induced and ICAM-1 is increased on local blood vessels, necessary for lymphocytes to move across the vessel wall. 4. Cytotoxic CD8+ T cells stimulated. 5. Chemokines including RANTES and MCP-1 attract a band of cytotoxic T cells which react with MHC class I on basal keratinocyte. TNF-α and IF-γ also induce ICAM-1 to be expressed on keratinocytes thus facilitating the migration of CD8+ lymphocytes into the epithelium. 6. Basal keratinocyte undergoes apoptosis.

inflammatory cells believed to be involved in the process include T helper (CD4+) and T cytotoxic (CD8+) lymphocytes, natural killer cells, and dendritic cells. The proposed sequence of events is shown in **Figure 1.2** whereby self-peptides are expressed and upregulated on the surface of keratinocytes. Langerhans's cells are recruited ultimately leading to clonal expansion of cytotoxic T cells with the help of T helper (CD4+) cells and IL12. Infiltration of cytotoxic T-cells in the epithelium leads to apoptosis of the basal keratinocytes. Possible mechanisms for apoptosis of keratinocytes include (1) TNF-α secreted by T cells binding to the TNF-α1 receptor on keratinocytes, (2) expression of $CD_{95}L$ (Fas ligand) on the surface of T cells, binding to CD_{95} (Fas) on the surface of keratinocytes and (3) cytotoxic T cells or NK cells releasing perforin which makes holes in the keratinocyte cell membrane and through which granzyme B secreted by T cells leads to cell death [10]. In addition, pro-inflammatory chemokines such as RANTES are produced by T lymphocytes, keratinocytes and mast cells among other cells. Several cell surface receptors for RANTES, e.g. CCR_1, CCR_3 CCR_4 CCR_5, CCR_9, CCR_{10} have been identified in OLP. RANTES can attract mast cells which then degranulate and release TNF-α and more chemokines, further stimulating RANTES. This cycle has been implicated in disease chronicity. In susceptible individuals chronic presentation of antigen may perpetuate the condition [11].

CLINICAL PRESENTATION OF OLP

Idiopathic OLP is a symmetrical condition in contrast to an irritant or contact lichenoid reaction which is often asymmetrical. While patients typically present with a variety of clinical features, distinct patterns are recognised and the terminology can be helpful to describe features in individual cases (**Table 1.1**) [12,13]. Lichen planus results in a dysregulation of keratinocyte turnover so that areas may be thickened, thinned or

Table 1.1 Clinical subtypes with frequency in oral lichen planus [12,13].	
Type	Frequency
Reticular	92%
Atrophic	44%
Plaque-type	36%
Papular	11%
Ulcerative	6%
Bullous	1%

ulcerated. Thus clinical subtypes include reticular, papular, plaque, atrophic, bullous and ulcerative subtypes (see **Figure 1.3**). The atrophic, bullous and ulcerative forms may lead to significant morbidity with discomfort during eating, swallowing or speech. The most commonly affected sites are the buccal mucosa, tongue and gingivae. The severity of OLP is broad ranging from mild and asymptomatic to severe, chronic, painful and ultimately leading to potential scarring. Approximately, 15% of patients with OLP go on to develop cutaneous lesions within several months of the initial onset of oral lesions.

Reticular OLP

The reticular form is the most common oral presentation frequently involving the buccal mucosa, lips, tongue or gingivae. While the majority of the patients are asymptomatic some may complain of roughness or dryness of the affected areas [14]. It presents as a white, linear or lacy pattern known as Wickham's striae. Within the reticular lesions, erythematous (atrophic) and ulcerative areas may develop (**Figure 1.3**).

Atrophic and ulcerative OLP

Atrophic lesions are common (44%) appearing as symptomatic erythematous areas and patients often report intolerance to spicy or acidic foods. When affecting the dorsum of the tongue, the lateral margins are affected initially leading to a hemilunar depapillation often with sparing of the lingual tip. Once lost the papillae do not reappear leaving a smooth atrophic surface. Within atrophic areas, progressive inflammation may lead to ulceration. Disease activity will fluctuate and most frequently affects the buccal mucosa, ventrolateral aspects of the tongue, gingivae and occasionally the lips. It is these patients that tend to present to dermatology clinics and where topical treatments fail to control symptoms, systemic therapy may be needed (see management algorithm).

Desquamative gingivitis

Gingival LP may be mild and appear as a glassy erythema with or without lichenoid striae or may progress to form areas of desquamation or frank ulceration known as desquamative gingivitis (DG) (see **Figure 1.3c**). Patients with DG may also be at risk of developing the VVG-LP sub-type or rarely in males peno-gingival LP. As seen in **Figures 1.4a** and **b** gingival LP may progress to a keratotic appearance and ultimately to verrucous changes that must be biopsied. These patients need to be monitored as they have a higher risk of developing dysplastic changes or an oral squamous cell carcinoma.

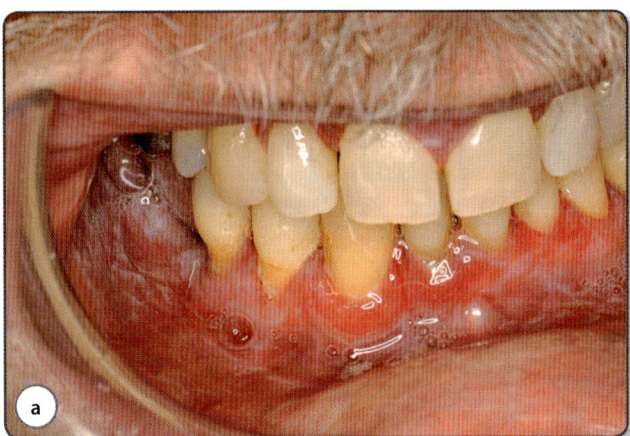

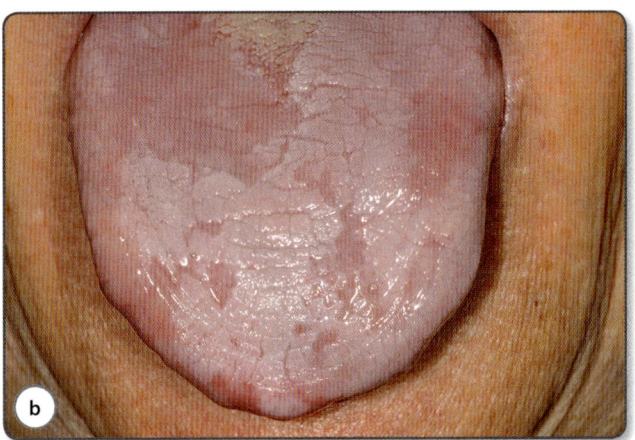

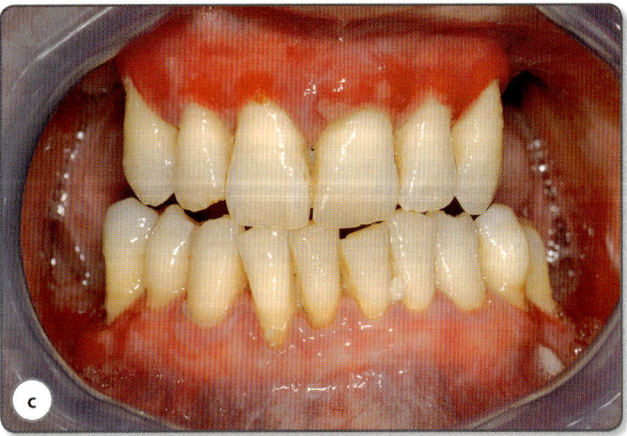

Figure 1.3 (a) Reticular striae present in the buccal sulcus and gingivae. Some background atrophic changes represented as erythema. (b) Papular lesions evolving into plaque type LP on the dorsum of the tongue. Papillae have been lost over most of the surface with central sparing. (c) Desquamative gingivitis with frank ulceration around upper incisors.

Papular and plaque OLP

Papular LP is typically seen on the dorsal aspect of the tongue or buccal mucosa as slightly elevated areas which may eventually become more homogeneous (Fig 1.3b) [15]. Plaque type lesions may present on any oral mucosal site. Most frequently they arise on the buccal mucosa or dorsum of tongue. Generally, a biopsy is advisable as the lesions are frequently asymmetrical and may represent an area of dysplasia arising within OLP. In some patients plaques may become progressively thickened with a verrucous appearance as seen in **Figure 1.4**.

Bullous OLP

Bullous OLP is rare. Patients will report a history of blisters but clinically the appearance is of typical OLP. The history may suggest an overlap with mucous membrane pemphigoid

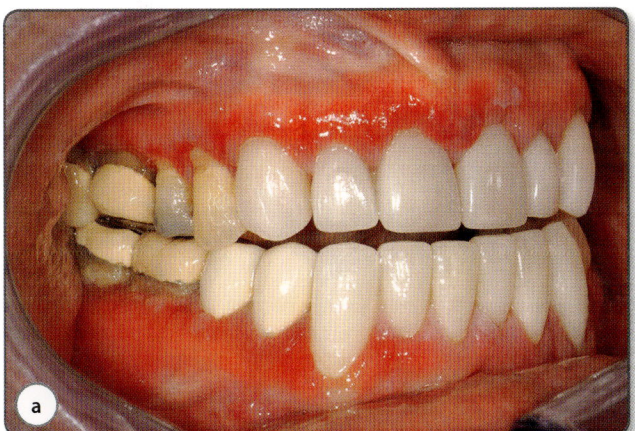

Figure 1.4 (a) Desquamative gingivitis with subtle keratotic changes on the gingiva. (b) 4 years later developing into verruccous hyperplasia.

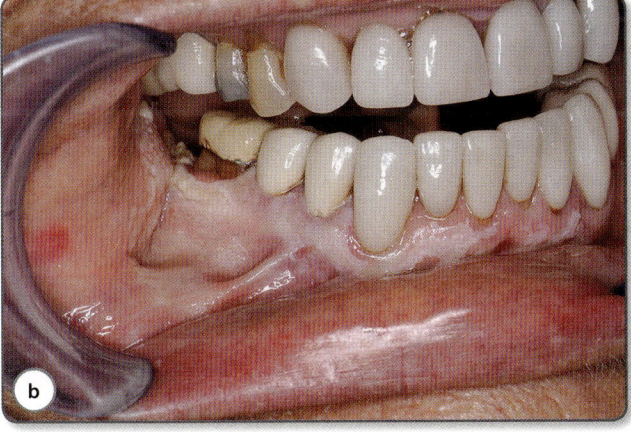

and a biopsy for histology and immunofluorescence is required for diagnosis. A ragged basement membrane zone fibrin band (Figure 1.1c) and absence of linear immunoglobulins or C3 is consistent with LP [2].

CLINICAL VARIANTS OF PREDOMINANTLY MUCOSAL LP

Oro-genital involvement

It is not unusual for patients to have other mucosal sites affected or to present with an oro-genital type of LP. In females the percentage with vulval LP is unknown but in a small series of 37 cases was 51% and may be associated with considerable morbidity [16]. Perianal involvement extending to the natal cleft may be present. In males, the penis similarly may be affected often with classical lichenoid papules or an erosive balanitis in approximately 5%.

The vulvovaginal gingival subtype of lichen planus

The VVG-LP is an uncommon and severe variant of LP characterised by erosions or desquamation of the vulval, vaginal and gingival mucosae which may heal with scarring. Patients may develop complications such as loss of vulval architecture, vaginal synechiae or stenosis [5]. Desquamative or ulcerative gingivitis is the most prominent oral manifestation and is essential for the diagnosis unless patients are edentulous, having lost their teeth due to severe gingival LP or being misdiagnosed as having chronic periodontitis. Extragingival sites may additionally be affected and intraoral scarring may be a prominent feature. Vertical fibrous bands occur in the buccal mucosae and result in a reduced oral aperture as well as loss of the buccal sulcal depth. This may lead to the appearance of the buccal mucosa being attached to the neck of the lower molars and functionally compromises tooth-brushing and oral hygiene. Patients frequently have other sites affected in this syndrome as demonstrated in **Figure 1.5**. Scarring in these sites is often prominent, e.g. oesophageal strictures, urethral strictures, lacrimal duct stenosis, scarring of the external ear canal, scarring alopecia and nail involvement. Therefore early recognition of VVG-LP and appropriate therapeutic

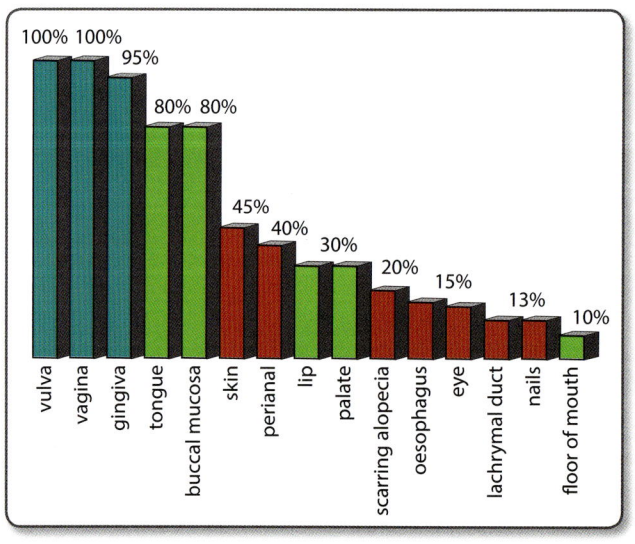

Figure 1.5 Sites of involvement in 40 patients with VVG-LP [5]. With permission from Journal of American Academy of Dermatology.

measures may help to reduce the significant physical and psychological morbidity associated with this scarring type of LP. In males there is a variant called peno-gingival LP. This is generally less severe than VVG as the penile lesions are very responsive to topical treatments and are generally recognised and treated at an earlier stage.

Extraoral mucosal sites may also be affected in OLP patients not fulfilling the criteria for VVG-LP. All of these cases require a multi-disciplinary approach to management. The association with ocular involvement is now well described but is still under-recognised. The most commonly affected site is the eyelid, which is the location of the lacrimal duct through which tears drains into the nose. Lacrimal canalicular obstruction results in epiphora secondary to overproduction of tears or inadequate drainage. Complications include conjunctival infections from stagnant tears and eczematous changes on the lower eyelid due to frequent tearing. Ocular LP may occasionally result in conjunctival inflammation and subepithelial fibrosis [17]. Other mucosal sites include the nose with symptoms of nasal crusting and erosions, and the oesophagus with patients having dysphagia. Oesophageal involvement may respond to immunosuppressive agents but often requires repeated oesophageal dilatations or stenting depending on the severity of the stricture formation.

Extraoral mucosal involvement

Cutaneous LP, present in 25% of OLP patients is typically a self-limiting condition and tends to resolve within 6–24 months though it can recur. Hypertrophic LP may be more persistent and may last for many years. Other persistent sites include the nails, scalp and external auditory canals, the latter being associated with scarring of the ear canal and may lead to conductive hearing loss.

Malignant potential in oral LP

Lichen planus is one of a group known as an oral potentially malignant disorder (OPMD). A systematic review of 16 studies determined a range of 0% to 3.5% for incidence [18]. While the data across studies is inconsistent with variations in diagnostic criteria, incomplete long-term follow up and lack of control populations an overall rate of malignancy is estimated to be 1.09%. There is a higher risk of transformation when lesions are present on the tongue, buccal mucosa or gingiva [18] and in patients with high risk behaviours such as smoking and excessive alcohol intake. In OLP, patients with an atypical clinical appearance particularly where the mucosa develops a firm or gritty texture, those with areas of ulceration that fail to respond to treatment and those with evolving plaque type LP particularly on the gingivae may warrant serial biopsies and close follow-up.

MANAGEMENT

Diagnosis

The diagnosis is confirmed following a detailed history including concurrent medication, other autoimmune diseases, a full clinical examination confirming symmetrical lesions and where indicated confirmatory histopathology and DIF.

There are important differential diagnoses to consider:

- Lichenoid reactions to dental materials are typically asymmetrical or unilateral LP-like lesion and are in direct contact with the relevant dental restoration. Reactions may be irritant or allergic and if required, patch testing may be undertaken though for a localised reaction removal of the restoration is usually recommended [19]

- Systemic medication may lead to oral or cutaneous lichenoid lesions and may be difficult to distinguish from idiopathic LP. The temporal association with a new medication may be helpful
- Discoid lupus erythematosus may lead to lichenoid lesions. They are relatively painless and may have a characteristic 'brush border'
- In patients with isolated DG without characteristic striae, immunobullous disorders such as pemphigus vulgaris or mucous membrane pemphigoid must be considered and investigated with DIF
- Finally plaque type LP, if isolated needs careful investigation and histopathology to confirm LP and exclude dysplasia

Assessment

Following a confirmed diagnosis, patients are examined for disease activity and overall severity. It is important to document carefully that each oral site has been examined enabling a more objective assessment of response to treatment over time. An oral disease

Table 1.2. Oral disease severity score (ODSS) (modified from Escudier [20].		
Site	Site score	Activity score (0–3) A score is allocated to each separate unit of site and these are added together
Outer lips (1)		
Inner lips (1)		
R Buccal mucosa (1 or 2) 1. <50% affected 2. >50% affected		
L Buccal mucosa (1 or 2)		
Gingivae (1 each segment)		
Lower R		
Lower central		
Lower L		
Upper R		
Upper central		
Upper L		
Dorsum of tongue (1 or 2)		
R Ventral tongue (1)		
L Ventral tongue (1)		
Floor of mouth (1 or 2)		
Hard palate (1 or 2)		
Soft palate (1 or 2)		
Oropharynx (1 or 2)		
Total		
Total Score = Site Score + Activity Score + Pain Score (1–10) (Maximum = 106)		

severity score (ODSS) devised and validated by the Oral Medicine Department at Guy's and St Thomas' Hospital in 2007 is one such method. (**Table 1.2**). Sequential scores will then help to inform management and the success or otherwise of interventions. Clinical photographs may also be helpful for monitoring suspicious areas as in **Figure 1.4**.

Site score
- 0 = no visible lesion;
- buccal mucosa 1 = <50% of affected and 2 = >50%;
- dorsum of tongue, floor of mouth, hard or soft palate or oropharynx: 1 = unilateral lesion 2 = bilateral lesions

Activity score
0   asymptomatic white lesions
1   mild erythema (glassy erythema or erythema localised to 3 mm along margins of teeth)
2   Marked erythema (full thickness gingivitis, extensive atrophy or oedema on non-keratinised mucosa)
3   Ulceration at this site

Pain score
Analogue scale from 0 (no discomfort) to 10 (the most severe pain they have encountered with this condition so far). The patient is asked to provide a score reflecting their pain/discomfort as an average during the preceding week.

General measures
Maintenance of a high standard of oral hygiene is paramount as accumulation of plaque aggravates mucosal inflammation. Antiseptic mouthwashes such as 0.2% chlorhexidine digluconate (Corsodyl mouthwash or spray) twice weekly or 1.5% hydrogen peroxide 10 mL daily (e.g. Peroxyl TM mouthwash Colgate-Palmolive) may be helpful. It is also important to recognise and treat candida as this can further exacerbate symptoms in OLP. Recognition of possible irritant or contact allergic reactions such as from amalgam fillings may necessitate dental treatment and/or patch testing [2]. Once an assessment has been made as to the need or otherwise for treatment, a sequence of interventions may be considered (see **Figure 1.6**). Asymptomatic OLP requires no treatment and if the pattern is typical, patients may be reassured and discharged to their general dental practitioner for follow-up.

TOPICAL THERAPY
In symptomatic patients anti-inflammatory oral rinses or sprays containing benzydamine hydrochloride (e.g. Difflam 3M) or lignocaine gel may be used for analgesia. In 2011 a Cochrane review of OLP found no randomised controlled clinical trials (RCTs) that compared topical corticosteroids with placebo in patients with symptomatic OLP. Thus, the authors concluded that there was no evidence that one steroid is any more effective than another [21]. In a later Cochrane review (2012) of erosive LP, there was weak evidence that 0.025% clobetasol propionate lipid-loaded microspheres significantly reduce pain compared to conventional ointment in a study of 50 participants [22].

In practice, topical corticosteroids are considered the mainstay of initial treatment and betamethasone sodium phosphate 0.5 mg in 10 mL water as a 3-minute rinse and

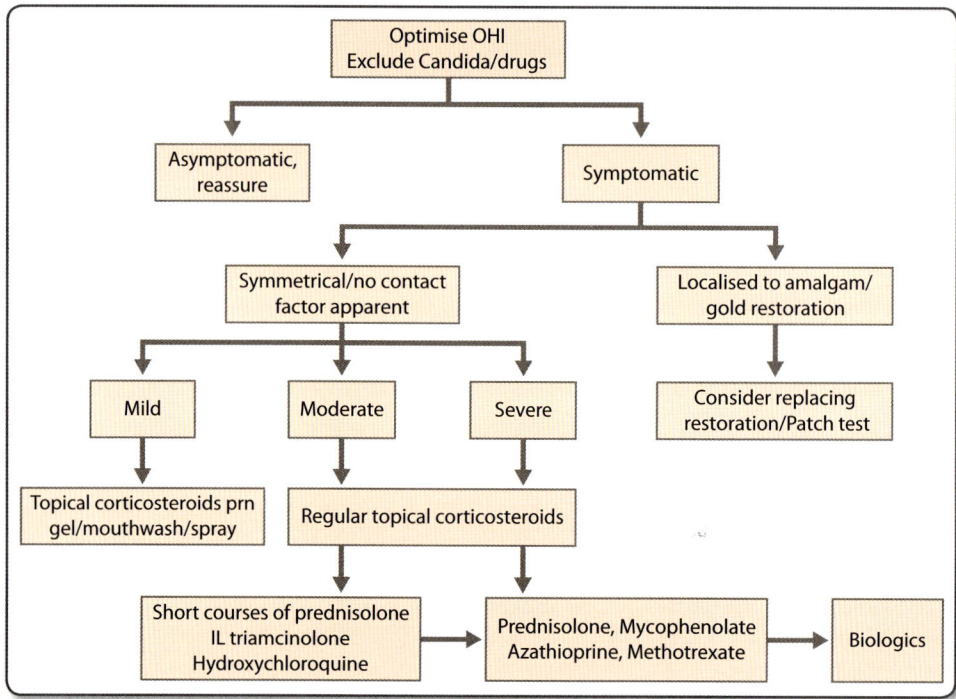

Figure 1.6 Algorithm for the management of oral lichen planus.

spit preparation up to four times daily (UCB Pharma Ltd, Watford, UK) or fluticasone propionate nasules (400 µg nasules in 10 mL water) twice daily may be helpful. For localized lesions clobetasol – 17-propionate 0.05% mixed in equal amounts with Orabase (ConvaTec, Uxbridge, UK) applied directly to the sulci, labial or buccal mucosae or within close fitting special trays may be helpful. If used frequently and long term, monitoring for adrenal suppression is recommended. The Cochrane review found weak evidence that aloe vera may reduce the pain of OLP and improve the clinical signs of disease compared to placebo. There was weak and unreliable evidence that topical Ciclosporin solution reduced pain compared to 0.1% triamcinolone acetonide. While nonrandomised studies have shown efficacy with topical tacrolimus the Cochrane review found no evidence for reduced pain compared to either steroids or placebo. Furthermore long-term safety is still to be determined and therefore, this is used only in short courses. The authors have found this very helpful for atrophic or erosive lesions on the lips used up to twice daily for 6 weeks avoiding strong sunlight during treatment.

Second line treatment

There is no consensus for an approach to second-line therapy. Intralesional corticosteroid preparations (5–10 mg/mL triamcinolone acetonide) once or twice weekly and repeated for 3–4 weeks may be used for localised ulceration. Thereafter the authors recommend a step-wise approach as detailed in **Figure 1.6**. Short courses of systemic steroids may be administered for rapid control of symptoms. Steroid-sparing agents, such as azathioprine, mycophenolate mofetil, methotrexate or ciclosporin, can be used with some evidence to support efficacy but there are no RCTs. Additionally systemic retinoids, antimalarials, dapsone, psoralen + UVA treatment (PUVA) and thalidomide have all been used with varied success. In our own clinical practice, favoured second approaches include short courses of prednisolone and/or hydroxychloroquine 200–400 mg daily. We would advocate consideration of this treatment in patients not yet requiring or not wishing to take immunosuppressive therapy [23]. Our data have shown improvement in ODSS scores in 18/43 (42%) patients by 3 months and 24/43 (56%) by 6 months. For recalcitrant oral lesions, or in severe cases of mucocutaneous LP, mycophenolate mofetil has been helpful when all other second line agents had failed [24].

Third line treatments

There is emerging evidence to suggest that biologics may be of benefit particularly when targeting TNF. In a recent literature review, Adalimumab successfully cleared a patient with oral and cutaneous LP in six weeks while in an OLP there was improvement with etanercept. While efalizumab and alefacept have also been associated with improvement they have both been withdrawn. Rituximab has been successful in one further patient with mucocutaneous LP [25]. Finally preliminary evidence is emerging to support the novel phosphodiesterase type IV inhibitor, apremilast in mucocutaneous LP.

FOLLOW-UP

Patients with symptomatic disease will require regular follow-up in secondary care, usually in an oral medicine department or in a combined oral dermatology setting. Patients on immunosuppressive agents will require 3-monthly blood tests and sequential disease severity scoring. The World Health Organisation has classified OLP as a premalignant condition. Therefore, patients with a diagnosis of OLP and either atypical or symptomatic disease should be informed of the low risk of cancer development and be monitored appropriately.

CONCLUSION

In summary the pathogenesis of mucosal LP is complex involving antigen presentation by oral keratinocytes leading to targeted inflammation and apoptosis of the basal epithelium. As these pathways are further elucidated, so more targeted therapies will emerge. In the meantime, it is important that clinicians recognise patients that require careful monitoring by a specialist MDT or oral medicine team. It is also important that they appreciate the scarring potential of mucosal LP particularly where patients have VVG-LP, ocular, oesophageal or otic disease, as early intervention may reduce the complication and associated morbidity.

Key points for clinical practice

- There is a strong association between OLP and thyroid disorders therefore check relevant personal/family history and consider undertaking thyroid function and a thyroid autoantibody screen.
- Consider the possibility of drug induced oral lichenoid changes and ascertain timing of addition of any new relevant medications.
- When patients present with gingival erythema or ulceration (DG) always check for the VGS as early detection and treatment will help to prevent serious scarring sequelae.

- Always consider possible dysplastic or malignant change in non-healing ulcers, progressive verrucous hyperplasia or firm white thickened nodules or plaques.
- Always arrange for a diagnostic biopsy before starting systemic therapy as this will confirm the diagnosis and indicate whether the patient has evidence of dysplasia.
- If patients develop a persistent new ulcer, a verrucous appearance to the mucosa or a firm keratotic lesion, refer to oral medicine or a maxillofacial surgery unit for a biopsy as malignancy develops in approximately 1:200 patients per year.
- If the patient has burning discomfort or disproportionate pain despite an apparent clinical improvement, check for oral candida.
- To assess response to treatment in OLP, use an objective disease scoring methodology such as the ODSS.
- Start treatment with topical oral corticosteroid preparations for 3 months and assess response.
- Consider a trial of hydroxychloroquine before moving to systemic immunosuppression.

REFERENCES

1. Vincent P, Breathnach SM, Le Cleach L. Lichen Planus and Lichenoid Disorders. In: Griffiths C, Barker J, Bleiker T, Chalmers R, Creamer D. Rook's Textbook of Dermatology, 4 Volume Set. Wiley, 2016.
2. Setterfield JF, Black MM, Challacombe SJ. The management of oral lichen planus. Clin Exp Dermatol 2000; 25:176–182.
3. Greenberg MS. AAOM Clinical Practice Statement: Subject: Oral lichen planus and oral cancer. Oral Surg Oral Med Oral Pathol Oral Radiol 2016; 122:440–441.
4. Liu J, Ye Z, Maher JG, et al. Phenome-wide association study maps new diseases to the human major histocompatibility complex region. J Med Genet 2016; 53:681–689.
5. Setterfield JF, Neill S, Shirlaw PJ, et al. The vulvovaginal gingival syndrome: A severe subgroup of lichen planus with characteristic clinical features and a novel association with the class II HLA DQB1*0201 allele. J Am Acad Dermatol 2006; 55:98–113.
6. Kurago Z. Aetiology and pathogenesis of oral lichen planus: an overview, Oral Surg Oral Med Oral Pathol Oral Radiol 2016; 122:72–80.
7. Chung PI, Hwang CY, Chen YJ, et al. Autoimmune comorbid diseases associated with lichen planus: A nationwide case-control study. J Eur Acad Dermatol Venereol 2015; 29:1570–1575.
8. Robledo-Sierra J, Mattsson U, Jontell M. Use of systemic medication in patients with oral lichen planus-a possible association with hypothyroidism. Oral Dis 2013; 19:313–319.
9. Thornhill MH, Sankar V, Xu XJ, et al. The role of histopathological characteristics in distinguishing amalgam-associated oral lichenoid and oral lichen planus. J Oral Pathol Med 2006; 35:233–240.
10. Thornhill MH. The current understanding of the aetiology of oral lichen planus. Oral Diseases 2010; 16:507–508.
11. Nogueira PA, Carneiro S, Ramos-e-Silva M. Oral lichen planus: an update on its pathogenesis Int Dermatol 2015; 54:1005–1010.
12. Andreasen JO. Oral lichen planus 1. A clinical evaluation of 115 cases. Oral Surg Oral Med Oral Pathol 1968; 25:31–42.
13. Thom JJ, Holmstrup P, Rindum J, Pindborg JJ. Course of various clinical forms of oral lichen planus. A prospective follow-up study of 611 patients. J Oral Pathol 1988; 17:213–218.
14. Ion DI, Setterfield JF. Oral Lichen Planus. Prim Dent J 2016; 5:40–44.
15. Van Der Waal J. Oral Lichen planus. In: Slootweg P. Dental and oral pathology. Switzerland: Springer Reference 2016:290–293.
16. Lewis FM, Shah M, Harrington CI. Vulval involvement in lichen planus: a study of 37 women. Br J Dermatol 1996; 135:89.
17. Webber NK, Setterfield JF, Lewis FM, et al. Lacrimal canalicular duct scarring in patients with lichen planus. Arch Dermatol 2012; 148:224–227.

18. Fitzpatrick SG, Hirsch SA, Gordon SC. The malignant transformation of oral lichen planus and oral lichenoid lesion: a systematic review J Am Dental Assoc 2014; 145:45–56.

19. Thornhill MH, Pemberton MW, Simmons RK, Theaker ED. Amalgam contact hypersensitivity lesions and oral lichen planus. Oral Surg Oral Med Oral Path 2003; 95:291–299.

20. Escudier M, Ahmed A, Shirlaw PJ, et al. A scoring system for assessing Oral Mucosal Diseases: Application to oral lichen planus. Br J Dermatol 2007; 157:765–770.

21. Thongprasom K, Carrozzo M, Furness S, Lodi G. Interventions for treating oral lichen planus. Cochrane Database Syst Rev 2011:CD001168.

22. Cheng S, Kirtschig G, Cooper S, et al. Interventions for erosive lichen planus affecting mucosal sites. Cochrane Database Syst Rev 2012:CD008092.

23. McParland H, Momen SE, Ormond M, et al. Efficacy of hydroxychloroquine in 43 patients with oral lichen planus (abstr). Oral Dis 2016; 22:14.

24. Wee JS, Shirlaw PJ, Challacombe SJ, Setterfield JF. Efficacy of mycophenolate mofetil in severe mucocutaneous lichen planus: a retrospective review of 10 patients. Br J Dermatol 2012; 167: 36–43.

25. Olsen MA, Rogers RS, Bruce AJ. Oral Lichen planus. Clin Dermatol 2016; 34:495–504.

Chapter 2

Morphoea management: current approaches and future perspectives

Amanda M Saracino Catherine H Orteu

INTRODUCTION

To date, our approach to managing patients with morphoea has been largely untargeted, with broad suppression of inflammation and sclerosis, and the exploitation of often serendipitously identified and poorly understood drug effects. However, as we begin to recognise the clinical heterogeneity of morphoea, and unravel the potential underlying molecular immunopathogenic determinants of disease subsets, the development of targeted treatments with a precise therapeutic rationale is becoming a realistic goal.

This chapter will briefly set out an up to date clinical approach to morphoea, describe the evidence base, rationale and strategies for the use of currently available treatments, and discuss future therapeutic targets based on our increasing understanding of disease mechanisms.

CLINICALLY GUIDED TREATMENT DECISIONS

Treatment decisions in morphoea must be guided by disease severity, which should in turn reflect clinical subtype, level of disease activity, degree of potential irreversible damage and patient focussed quality of life (QoL) indices (see **Figure 2.1** and **2.2**) [1–5].

Morphoea classification is laden with inconsistency and has been largely based on anatomical disease distribution [4]. However, such approaches do not capture the clinical complexity of morphoea. Morphologically, varying degrees of inflammation, sclerosis, atrophy and/or dyspigmentation can occur both within and between individuals. Deep tissue involvement, beyond the dermis can occur in all subtypes of morphoea (most commonly linear and generalised). It frequently involves the subcutis and fascia, and more rarely underlying muscle, bone, eye and brain. When present, deep tissue involvement

Amanda M Saracino MBBS BMedSc FACD, University College London, Royal Free Campus and Royal Free London NHS Foundation Trust, London, UK

Catherine H Orteu BSc MD FRCP, University College London, Royal Free Campus and Royal Free London NHS Foundation Trust, London, UK. Email: cate.orteu@nhs.net (for correspondence)

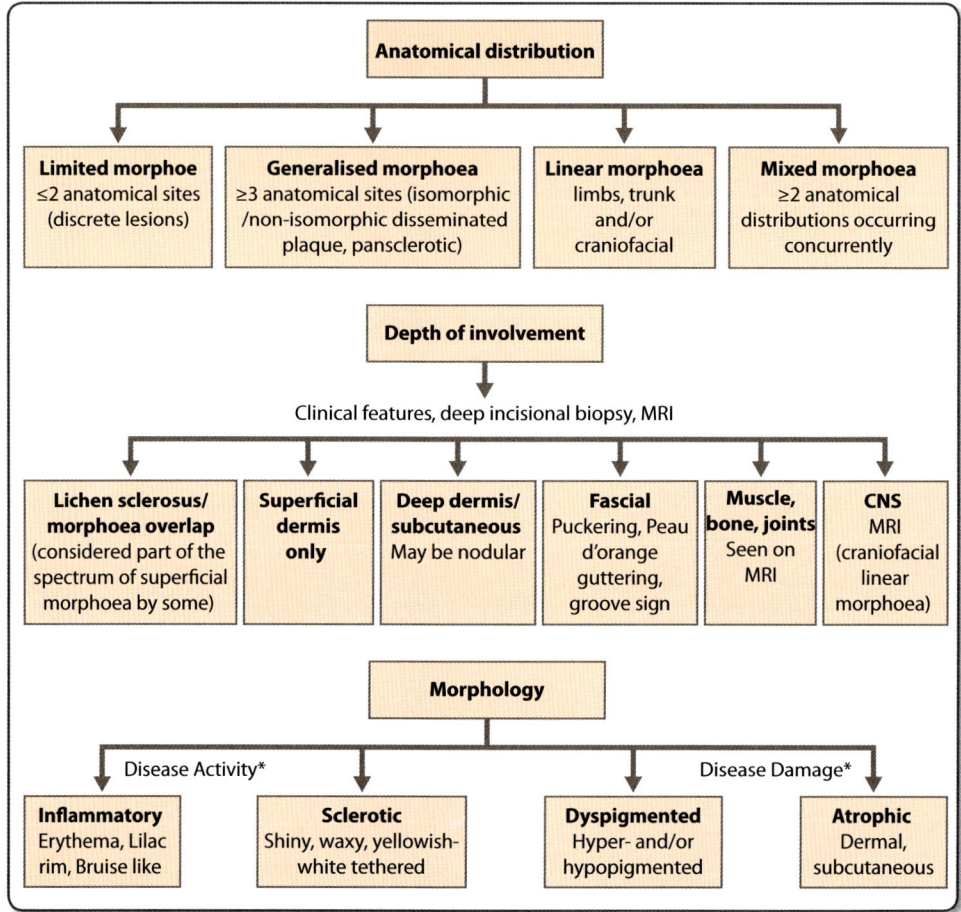

Figure 2.1A A three-tiered approach to clinical morphoea classification according to anatomical distribution/ patterning, depth of tissue involvement and clinical morphology.
*Inflammation and sclerosis generally reflect disease activity, whilst atrophy and dyspigmentation generally reflect disease damage. However, these clinical phases can occur concurrently in one individual and variably between individuals.

has important implications on morbidity and outcomes. Hence a three-tiered approach to morphoea classification, characterising all these disease aspects, has great clinical utility (see **Figure 2.1**) [6].

Objectively measuring disease activity, subsequent response to therapy and permanent damage remains challenging. A number of imaging techniques or histology may be utilised, however these methods can be expensive, highly specialised, time inefficient and not readily available [3,4,7,8]. Accordingly, the localised scleroderma cutaneous assessment tool (LoSCAT) is now increasingly used as a validated, practical, clinical measure of morphoea activity and damage, which is responsive to change [9].

Finally, disease severity and treatment decisions in morphoea also depend on patient focussed disease morbidity. This is directly related to psychosocial impact, cosmetic and functional complications. Dermatology life quality index (DLQI) and the hospital anxiety

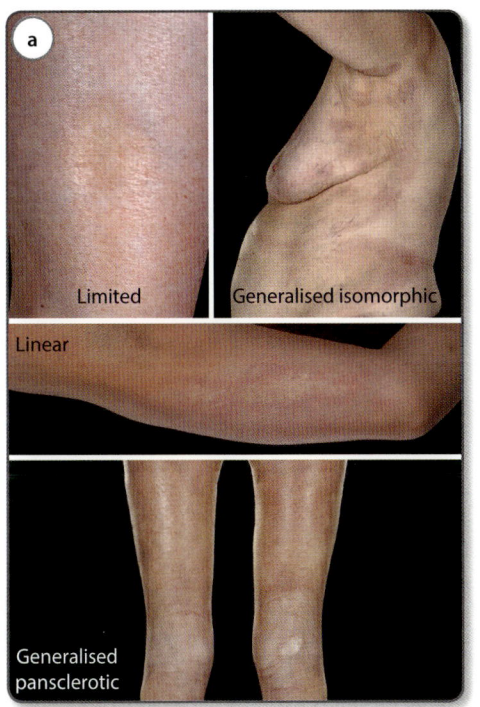

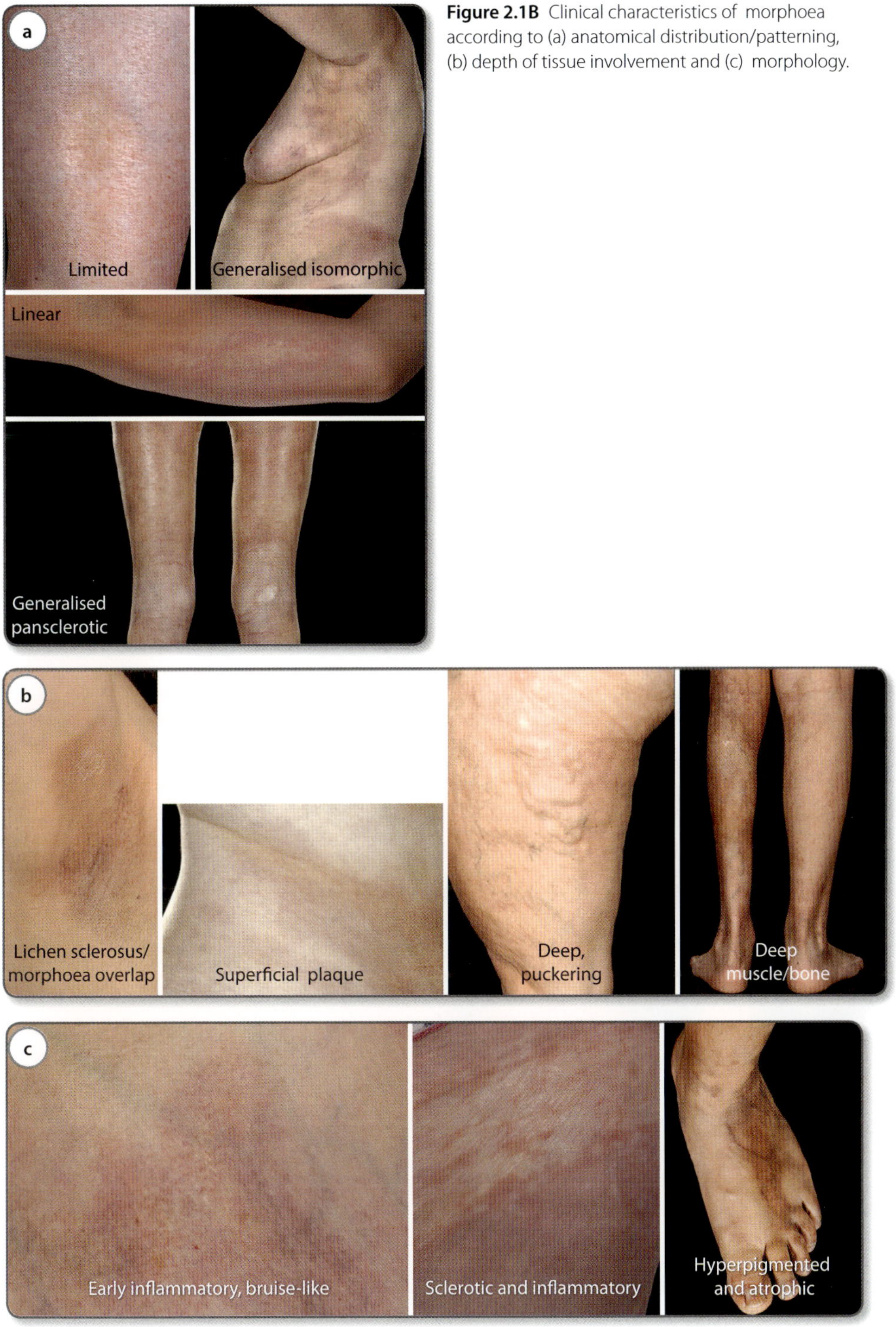

Figure 2.1B Clinical characteristics of morphoea according to (a) anatomical distribution/patterning, (b) depth of tissue involvement and (c) morphology.

a

Limited   Generalised isomorphic

Linear

Generalised pansclerotic

b

Lichen sclerosus/ morphoea overlap   Superficial plaque   Deep, puckering   Deep muscle/bone

c

Early inflammatory, bruise-like   Sclerotic and inflammatory   Hyperpigmented and atrophic

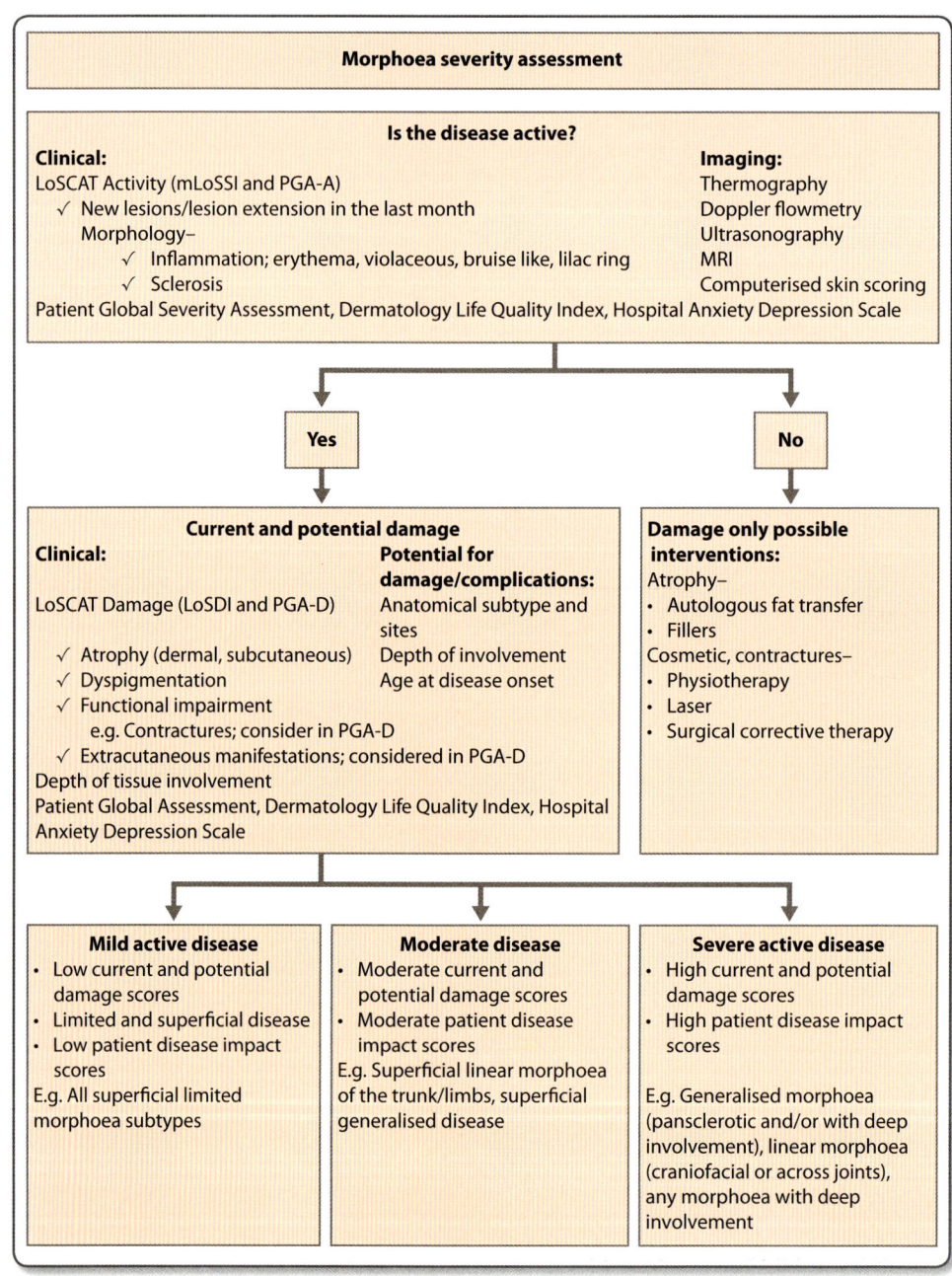

Figure 2.2 Clinically guided treatment decisions. A clinical approach to morphoea severity assessments, based on level of disease activity and damage; used to guide treatment decisions according to mild, moderate and severe disease.

LoSCAT = localised scleroderma cutaneous assessment tool, mLoSSI = modified localised scleroderma severity index (part of LoSCAT, activity score), LoSDI = localised scleroderma damage index (part of LoSCAT, damage score), PGA-A = physician global assessment of activity (part of LoSCAT), PGA-D = physician global assessment of damage (part of LoSCAT).

and depression scale (HADS) (or paediatric equivalents) can be utilised to monitor patient centred disease impact; with higher scores reported in linear and generalised disease [10,11].

Put together, baseline and serial assessments of disease severity are vital to ensuring appropriate treatment decisions. This must include consideration of markers of morphoea subtypes, disease activity, current and potential future damage, as well as patient focussed QoL indices (see **Figure 2.2**). Prompt and accurate identification of those at increased risk of complications, and early commencement of appropriate therapy are vital, if we are to minimise tissue damage and improve patient outcomes.

CURRENT TREATMENT APPROACHES

A number of topical, physical and systemic treatment options are available for morphoea and we will now consider the evidence for these (see **Table 2.1** and **Figure 2.3**) [1–3,8,12,13].

Topical therapies

Topical treatments can be useful and efficacious in limited forms of superficial inflammatory and/or sclerotic morphoea. In more widespread or severe subtypes, topical preparations can act as a potential adjunct, especially if symptoms (e.g. pruritus) are prominent at localised sites of superficial involvement. However widespread application is often impractical in generalised morphoea, and due to limited penetration topical therapies have minimal benefit in deep tissue involvement. Application under occlusion improves penetration and may improve efficacy in some settings.

Tacrolimus

Tacrolimus is a macrolide antibiotic which inhibits calcineurin, hence inhibiting several proinflammatory and profibrotic mediators, such as IL-2, tumour necrosis factor-alpha (TNF-α) and interferon-gamma (IFN-γ), known to be involved in skin sclerosis and morphoea pathogenesis.

Case reports, prospective uncontrolled and one controlled trial, have reported the application of tacrolimus 0.1% ointment in 31 morphoea patients; 30 with limited plaque and one with disseminated plaque subtypes. This literature supports the twice daily application of tacrolimus 0.1% ointment for 3–4 months (either under occlusion, or not), with significant improvements noted in clinical and histological outcome measures in the majority of cases. Active inflammatory lesions, with or without accompanying mild to moderate sclerotic change, appear most responsive.

Vitamin D analogues

Calcipotriene and calcipotriol are analogues of vitamin D available in topical preparations. Importantly, they inhibit fibroblast proliferation and collagen synthesis, and exposure of morphoea fibroblasts to calcipotriol results in a 20-fold inhibition of cell proliferation. Vitamin D analogues also have well recognised effects on keratinocyte proliferation and differentiation, and the relevance of this in morphoea is of interest, as the role of keratinocytes in skin fibrosis is increasingly documented.

The efficacy of topical calcipotriol or calcipotriene 0.005% has been demonstrated in case reports, one case series and two prospective uncontrolled studies, either as solitary therapy applied twice daily under occlusion for at least 3 months to plaque or linear morphoea (13 patients), with betamethasone dipropionate applied once or twice daily to active plaque morphoea (7 patients) or in combination with low dose ultraviolet A1 (UVA-1) phototherapy in 19 children.

Immiquimod

Imiquimod is an imidazoquinolone; a class of immunoenhancing drugs that mobilise cytokines. The mechanism of action of imiquimod in morphoea is somewhat of a conundrum, however it has been hypothesised that as an IFN-γ inducer, it can inhibit Connective tissue growth factor-beta (TGF-β); a key orchestrator of sclerosis. Also of potential relevance are the antiangiogenic effects of imiquimod, once again via IFN-γ induction.

Evidence supports the use of 5% imiquimod cream in morphoea, applied 3–7 times weekly for between 6 weeks and 9 months. Most recently, a placebo-controlled trial of 22 patients showed statistically significant improvements in induration (best demonstrated improvement), size and dyspigmentation at 3, 6 and 9 months. Local irritation and ulceration occurred in 24% of this cohort. Shorter 6-week duration therapy has also previously resulted in improvement in size, erythema and induration of morphoea.

Topical corticosteroids

Topical corticosteroid preparations are the most commonly used therapy for limited plaque morphoea [3], are the most commonly used topical therapy overall by paediatric rheumatologists and in a recent survey of UK physicians, were rated amongst the most successful treatment modalities [14]. In practice, topical corticosteroids appear to be particularly effective in active inflammatory lesions, and those with associated epidermal change. However, no studies have specifically investigated the efficacy of topical corticosteroids in morphoea.

Of note, intralesional 5–10% triamcinolone, injected 4–6 weekly for 3–6 months, has shown mixed results in case reports and small series of 'en coup de sabre', nodular and limited plaque morphoea.

Physical therapies

Phototherapy

The mechanisms of action of phototherapy in morphoea are complex. Direct cellular effects include induction of T-cell apoptosis (immunohistochemistry of morphoea skin reveals significant reductions in T-cell markers on post-UVA treatment), depletion of mast cells, and of epidermal and dermal Langerhan cells. This affects inflammatory and profibrotic signalling pathways and cytokines. UVA mediated induction of collagen-degrading matrix metalloproteinases (MMPs; such as MMP-1, MMP-3, MMP-9 and possibly MMP-12) is well documented, and collagenase activity appears to correlate to UVA dose in morphoea. In addition, UVA can up-regulate haem-oxygenase-1, which has known antifibrotic effects. Importantly, signalling and levels of TGF-β are altered by UV-irradiation and this, as well as IFN-γ induction and IL-6 inhibition, correlate with the degree of phototherapy-induced skin softening.

Robust evidence for the clinical efficacy of phototherapy in morphoea is lacking, with variable dosing regimens and outcome measures making interpretation of the limited data extremely challenging [2,3,8,13,15,16]. Furthermore, very few studies compare different phototherapy modalities. However, UVA1 (340–400 nm), broadband (bb) UVA with or without topical or systemic psoralen (320–400 nm) and narrowband (nb) UVB (311 nm), have been utilised in the management of all types of morphoea, both in paediatric and adult populations, with at least some degree of success. For superficial limited or generalised morphoea, phototherapy may be tried before systemic treatments in appropriate cases (see **Table 2.1**, **Figures 2.2** and **2.3**). Importantly, longer wavelengths (namely UVA-1) penetrate more deeply than shorter wavelength phototherapy (e.g. bbUVA and nbUVB), but still do not reach beyond the dermis; potentially precluding their use in patients with deeper tissue involvement. Interestingly, however, rare cases of eosinophilic fasciitis have been successfully treated with UVA-1 and psoralen and ultraviolet A (PUVA), suggesting an indirect effect on deeper tissues.

With regards to clinical morphology, active inflammatory and/or sclerotic lesions appear to respond better to phototherapy than atrophic and/or dyspigmented lesions [2]. To date however, no studies have addressed this question directly.

UVA-1 phototherapy

Although inaccessibility often limits its utility, UVA-1 is the most widely studied form of phototherapy in morphoea and its efficacy has been demonstrated in two randomised controlled trials (RCTs) and several prospective studies. All doses (low; 10–20 J/cm^2, medium; >20–70 J/cm^2 and high; >70–120 J/cm^2) are beneficial, and although high dose may be most effective, the associated greater cumulative UV exposure makes it less preferable. When considering clinical outcome measures only (objective skin scores and visual analogue scale symptom scores), medium (40 treatments of 50 J/cm^2 or 30 treatments of 70 J/cm^2) and low (30–40 treatments of 20 J/cm^2) dose UVA-1 for 8–10 weeks are equally efficacious. Further support for low dose UVA-1 lies in its enhanced therapeutic efficacy when combined with topical application of vitamin-D analogues; this should be especially considered in cases where minimising cumulative UV exposure is important. However, medium dose (70 J/cm^2) UVA-1 is superior to low dose when the more sensitive end point of ultrasound skin thickness is utilised.

Duration of response to UVA-1 phototherapy in morphoea is variable, and although poorly studied, recurrent disease may occur in up to 45% of patients at 2–3 years, particularly in those individuals with more longstanding disease.

Interestingly, skin darkening resulting from UVA-1 treatment may attenuate its antifibrotic effects, suggesting phototherapy may be less effective in dark skinned individuals. However this remains controversial and a retrospective study found UVA-1 equally effective in 47 morphoea patients of different skin-phototypes.

Overall, where available, UVA-1 phototherapy should be first line in those requiring and suitable for phototherapy. Recommendations suggest medium doses (40–60 J/cm^2) 3–5 times weekly, for a total of 30–40 sessions, as the best balance of safety and efficacy (see **Table 2.1**).

UVA phototherapy; broadband and photochemotherapy

Limited evidence supports the use of bbUVA (with or without topical or systemic psoralen) in morphoea, and its accessibility in everyday dermatological practice makes resultant

Table 2.1 Evidence-based clinical recommendations for currently available morphoea treatments	
TREATMENT	**RECOMMENDED TREATMENTS**
Topical Therapy	
Tacrolimus 0.1% ointment	• Twice daily application, under occlusion if possible, for 3 months to active superficial inflammatory morphoea, with or without mild to moderate sclerosis
Calcipotriol 0.005% ointment	• Once or twice daily application under occlusion if possible, for at least 3 months to active superficial inflammatory and/or sclerotic morphoea, alone or in combination with betamethasone diproprionate • Combination therapy may enhance low dose UVA-1 efficacy
Imiquimod	• Thrice weekly to daily application, for 6 weeks–9 months in superficial morphoea with sclerosis, erythema and/or dyspigmentation • Patients must be warned regarding local irritation and possible ulceration, which may occur in up to one quarter of cases
Potent corticosteroids	• Once or twice daily application to active superficial inflammatory morphoea and/or lesions with overlying surface epidermal change
Physical Therapy	
Phototherapy	• Where available, medium dose (40–60 J/cm2) 3 to 5 times weekly UVA-1 phototherapy, for a total of 30–40 treatments, should be first line in those with superficial limited plaque morphoea unresponsive to topical treatments, or superficial generalised or linear (trunk/limbs) morphoea • Where UVA-1 is inaccessible, 3 times weekly PUVA (preferably bath/topical) for 30 treatments should be considered as a useful alternative • Where UVA-1 and PUVA are not available, 3 to 5 times weekly nbUVB for 40 treatments or 3 times weekly low to medium dose bbUVA for 20–30 treatments may be considered
Systemic therapy	
Methotrexate +/− corticosteroids	• Methotrexate, with or without corticosteroids, should be considered first line therapy for severe active morphoea • Combination systemic corticosteroids are of particular benefit in cases of inflammatory disease, and where there is deep subdermal involvement; the latter appears to be particularly steroid responsive • Treatment duration of 2–4 years is recommended, to potentially minimise disease recurrence, which can occur many years post-treatment
Mycophenolate mofetil	• In morphoea requiring systemic therapy, MMF should be considered as 2nd line to MTX, or 1st line in cases where MTX is contraindicated; with corticosteroids especially in the setting of inflammatory disease and/or subdermal deep involvement • Combination MTX and MMF may be useful if monotherapy has failed or is contraindicated
Hydroxychloroquine	• Hydroxychloroquine has antifibrotic affects in vitro and may be a useful add-on therapy in some cases • Hydroxychloroquine may be a useful adjunct for extracutaneous manifestations such as arthralgia, arthritis, myalgia and fatigue seen in up to one-third of patients with linear and generalised disease • Hydroxychloroquine may lessen skin tenderness in morphoea
Ciclosporin	• The evidence for ciclosporin in morphoea is limited, with single case reports suggesting its possible use, especially in generalised disease with deep involvement
Abatacept/tocilizumab	• Abatacept and pocilizumab are supported by limited case reports in morphoea, and further cases of systemic sclerosis, but are limited by affordability and accessibility

Treatment of active morphoea by disease severity		
Mild	**Moderate**	**Severe**
✓ Low current and potential Damage Scores ✓ Low patient disease impact scores *Classification subtypes:* ✓ Superficial limited disease **First Line:** Topicals (8-12 week trial) 2a - Tacrolimus Imiquimod 2b- Calcipotriol +/- Betamethasone 3 - Corticosteroids **Second Line:** Phototherapy (30-40 treatments) 1b- UVA1 (1st line where available) nbUVB (3rd line) 2b–PUVA (2nd line where UVA-1 not accessible)	✓ Moderate current and potential Damage Scores ✓ Moderate patient disease impact scores *Classification subtypes:* ✓ Superficial generalised morphoea (eg. disseminated plaque) ✓ Superficial linear morphoea of the trunk or limbs (adult onset) **First Line:** Topicals (8-12 week trial) 2a - Tacrolimus Imiquimod 2b- Calcipotriol +/- Betamethasone 3 - Corticosteroids *And* Phototherapy (30-40 treatments) 1b- UVA1 (1st line where available) nbUVB (3rd line) 2b–PUVA (2nd line where UVA-1 not accessible)	✓ High current and potential Damage Scores ✓ High patient disease impact scores ✓ Mild to moderate morphoea failing to respond to therapy (or contraindicated) +/- with high patient disease impact scores *Classification subtypes:* ✓ Generalised morphoea (especially pansclerotic or deep disseminated plaque) ✓ Craniofacial linear morphoea ✓ Linear morphoea of the trunk / limbs with deep involvement and / or paediatric onset ✓ Limited morphoea with deep involvement **First Line:** 1b - MTX +/- IV or oral CS **Second Line:** 3 - MMF +/ IV or oral CS **Third Line:** 3 -Combine MTX + MMF Combine systemic + phototherapy Combine with HCQ **Fourth Line:** 3 - Abatacept, Tocilizumab (limited by accessibility) Ciclosporin ECP Other experimental and reported therapies
Level of Evidence: 1a – meta-analysis of RCT 1b – at least one RCT 2a – at least one controlled study 2b – at least one other type of quasi-controlled study 3 – non-experimental descriptive studies 4 – expert opinion		

Figure 2.3 Treatment options for active morphoea according to disease severity, with supported level of evidence (1a to 4).

recommendations more clinically applicable. A total of 101 patients have been treated with bbUVA alone in the literature [three prospective studies (one controlled) and two case reports], showing >50% clinical improvements overall, with or without concurrent histological parameter improvements after 20 low (5 J/cm^2), medium (10 J/cm^2) or high (20 J/cm^2) dose treatments. There does not appear to be a significant difference between variable bbUVA dosing regimens.

More extensive case reports and small case series have demonstrated clinically significant improvements in adult and paediatric limited plaque, linear and generalised morphoea with systemic and topical (bath or cream) PUVA [16]. A further 62 patients have received PUVA (11 systemic, 47 bath and 4 cream) in prospective uncontrolled studies [16]. Treatment was twice to thrice weekly for up to 30 sessions, and at least 85% showed clinically significant improvement or complete clearance (with additional parameter improvements in some; such as ultrasound skin thickness or circulating immunological markers). Improvements tended to be seen by treatment 15 in most [16]. Whilst the evidence is difficult to make clear comparisons from, expert opinion favours the use of topical over systemic PUVA in morphoea.

Narrowband UVB phototherapy

Finally, although most readily available and easily employed, there is limited evidence for the use of nbUVB in morphoea, in keeping with its superficial dermal penetration. One randomised-controlled study demonstrated nbUVB (8 weeks, 40 treatments) was as effective as low dose (50 J/cm^2) UVA-1 of identical frequency and duration, but inferior to medium dose (50 J/cm^2) UVA-1. A further uncontrolled prospective study showed comparable improvements in clinical and ultrasound parameters for PUVA and nbUVB after 12 weeks (regimens not clear). Combination nbUVB (thrice weekly) with acitretin was effective in a single case of postirradiation (breast cancer) induced plaque morphoea.

Extracorporeal photopheresis

The benefits of extracorporeal photopheresis (ECP) are well established in diseases caused by aberrant T-lymphocytes, including cutaneous T-cell lymphoma and graft-versus-host disease (GvHD). Blood is removed, leukocytes are treated with photosensitising methoxsalen and subsequently exposed to UVA radiation. This results in apoptosis, predominantly of T-cells, but also B-cells, monocytes and natural killer cells. Apoptotic cells then inhibit the production of proinflammatory cytokines involved in fibrosis such as IL-1, IL-6 and TNF-α.

ECP is reported in over 100 patients with systemic sclerosis (SSc) or morphoea, with some positive outcomes [15]. This has included five cases of severe treatment resistant generalised morphoea, and a RCT of 44 patients with SSc, who showed statistically significant improvement in skin severity scores and joint contractures [15,17].

Laser

Likely mimicking phototherapy, monochromatic excimer laser (308 nm) may be helpful in improving skin texture and dyspigmentation in morphoea [18].

Pulsed dye laser (585 nm) has also been used with at least some success in several patients with limited plaque morphoea, producing improvements in skin texture and dyspigmentation. CD34+ fibrocytes are transformed to CD34– myofibroblasts in morphoea, with a subsequent increase in factor XIIIa expressing cells which enhance collagen and extracellular matrix production. PDL appears to reverse this, with increased CD34+ cells and decreased factor XIIIa expression seen on skin biopsy post-treatment.

Fractionated CO_2 laser has been successfully utilised in contractures occurring as a consequence of morphoea in a single case report. However, the possibility of impaired wound healing and theoretical risk of trauma induced disease reactivation must be considered.

SYSTEMIC THERAPIES

In cases of severe active morphoea, systemic therapy should be considered early to minimise morbidity and long-term permanent damage (see **Figures 2.2** and **2.3**). Methotrexate, often with corticosteroids, is now accepted as first line treatment in such cases; including craniofacial linear morphoea, linear morphoea of the limbs or trunk with deep involvement and/or crossing joints, generalised disease, or limited morphoea with deep involvement [1,8,19–24].

Corticosteroids

Corticosteroids, in the form of oral prednisolone and/or intravenous pulsed methylprednisolone (IVMP), have been utilised in isolation and as combination therapy. Although variable, typical dosing of oral prednisolone is 0.5–1 mg/kg (adults) or 1–2 mg/kg (children) for 1–3 months, weaning over 1–18 months (in isolation or as maintenance post-IVMP); and IVMP is 1 g weekly (adults) or 30 mg/kg weekly (children) for 3 consecutive weeks, or daily for 3 consecutive days per week, for up to 3–6 months [1].[1]

Considering the use of corticosteroids as monotherapy, an uncontrolled study of 17 patients with linear and generalised disease showed a 100% response rate (4 achieved complete resolution) to 0.5–1 mg/kg/day prednisolone for 6 weeks (subsequently weaned over 18 months); however 33% relapsed after treatment discontinuation.

Of note, systemic corticosteroids appear to be of particular benefit in the setting of deep involvement, with up to 94% of those classified as having eosinophilic fasciitis responding to steroids alone (oral and/or IVMP) [21]. Prompt resolution of early phase oedema is seen, with concurrent normalisation of ESR, peripheral eosinophilia and hypergammaglobulinaemia. Intravenous pulsed methylprednisolone appears to have additional effects, with more patients receiving both IVMP and oral corticosteroids achieving complete remission, and fewer requiring the subsequent addition of a steroid sparing immunosuppressive agent [21]. However relapse with corticosteroid monotherapy remains high even in cases of eosinophilic fasciitis, and hence most require concomitant immunosuppression [21,25].

Methotrexate

Methotrexate primarily inhibits dihydrofolate reductase, however, a variety of additional mechanisms are involved in its anti-inflammatory and antifibrotic effects in morphoea. Methotrexate inhibits T-cell activation, selectively down regulates B-cells and inhibits methyltransferase, leading to deactivation of immune related enzymatic activity. Of likely specific relevance to sclerotic skin disease, methotrexate can reduce serum tenascin, IL-2, IL-4, IL-6, IL-8 and soluble TNF-receptor levels, all of which have demonstrated potential roles in morphoea pathogenesis [6]. Additionally, methotrexate results in IL-1 receptor antagonisation, and the potential inciting role of keratinocyte-derived IL-1 in morphoea immunopathogenesis is recognised [6].

A number of retrospective [21,22], prospective [20,23,24,26] and one RCT [19] have evaluated the successful short- and long-term efficacy of methotrexate and combination methotrexate with corticosteroids, in paediatric and adult onset morphoea and eosinophilic fasciitis.

As monotherapy, methotrexate has efficacy (oral or subcutaneous, at doses from 15–25 mg weekly in adults, and 0.3–0.6 mg/kg in children) in plaque, linear and generalised morphoea [24]. Clinically significant responses are seen as early as 2 months and longevity of remission appears to relate to duration of treatment and cumulative dose achieved.

Combination corticosteroid and methotrexate therapy for active moderate to severe morphoea is supported by one RCT and appears to have advantages over either treatment as monotherapy [19]. Superficial (dermis only) disease may be more responsive to methotrexate [21], and methotrexate appears to lessen relapse rates by up to two-thirds [22]. However, the addition of corticosteroids may enable a more rapid treatment response, especially in those with recent onset, possibly more inflammatory, disease, and in the setting of deep, subdermal involvement [21]. Hence overall, combined treatment tends to be recommended [1,23].

Methotrexate treatment duration and disease relapse

Relapsing and chronically active morphoea occur frequently in both adults and children. Overall, average disease duration and relapse rates appear to be higher in childhood onset morphoea [27]; with 20% still active after 20 years and continuously active disease seen well into adulthood in 30%. Regardless of age of onset, disease recurrence is more frequent in linear morphoea of the limbs [27], and can occur even after many years of quiescence [1,27].

Post-treatment recurrence rates are reported in 15–65%, 16–24 months after cessation of methotrexate in children and adults [25,27], with up to 40% requiring further treatment courses after an average of 21 months off therapy [24]. However, recurrence rates appear to be inversely related to duration of methotrexate therapy and cumulative dose achieved. There is now mounting evidence to support longer treatment courses of 3–4 years [25].

Mycophenolate mofetil (MMF)

In addition to its immunosuppressive and anti-inflammatory effects, the antifibrotic properties of MMF are also documented and increasingly exploited. MMF can reduce or even abrogate fibroblast proliferation in response to proliferative stimuli by down regulating profibrotic cytokines and chemokines including TGFβ-1, Smad 2 and 3, CCL2/MCP-1 and IL-6, reducing profibrotic factor plasminogen activator inhibitor-1, thereby decreasing extracellular matrix components such as fibronectin and connective tissue growth factor (CTGF).

Unsurprisingly therefore, the efficacy of MMF in sclerotic diseases is increasingly reported [28], with antifibrotic effects on skin in SSc now well recognised [29]. MMF has demonstrated efficacy in plaque, linear and generalised morphoea, pansclerotic morphoea of childhood, and eosinophilic fasciitis; either alone, with MTX and/or corticosteroids, or in combination with PUVA. In those requiring systemic therapy, MMF is recommended as second line treatment by the Childhood Arthritis and Rheumatology Research Alliance (CARRA) (see **Table 2.1**) [1].

Of note, distinct genetic 'intrinsic subsets' in SSc have been described, with reproducible gene expression profiles correlating to inflammatory and fibroproliferative signatures. Gene expression profiles change pre- and post-treatment with MMF in those who demonstrate significant modified Rodnan skin thickness score (mRSS) improvements. Responses are seen in those of the inflammatory subset [30], and importantly, three morphoea patients have been linked to this genetic expression profile.

Hydroxychloroquine

Although cases of morphoea successfully treated with hydroxychloroquine have been reported for decades, the in vitro antifibrotic effects of this multifaceted drug are only recently being recognised. Primarily, hydroxychloroquine is an immunomodulator, with inhibitory effects on a variety of proinflammatory innate and adaptive immune pathways with potential roles in skin sclerosis; such as TLRs, IFN-γ, IL-1, TNF-α and Th17 related cytokines (IL-6, IL-17 and IL-22). Further, and of great potential relevance to morphoea, chloroquine suppresses basic-fibroblast growth factor (bFGF) and hydroxychloroquine induces autophagic cell death of human dermal fibroblasts. The latter reduces fibroblast metabolic activity and proliferation via decreased phosphorylation of profibrotic extracellular signal-regulated kinase-1 and 2 (ERK-1/2) [6].

Interestingly, a majority of documented responses to hydroxychloroquine have been in patients with eosinophilic fasciitis. Whether this reflects an increased responsiveness of deep morphoea and fasciitis to the drug's anti-inflammatory effects (paralleling the response to corticosteroids), rather than any direct antifibrotic effects of the drug per se, remains uncertain. A retrospective review of craniofacial linear morphoea, where most patients (7 of 11) treated with hydroxychloroquine showed no improvement supports this view. In contrast though, decreased dermal sclerosis in response to hydroxychloroquine monotherapy in morphoeaiform cutaneous sarcoidosis, and sclerodermic linear lupus panniculitis are reported, supporting hydroxychloroquine's direct in vivo antifibrotic effects.

Finally, hydroxychloroquine can reduce constitutional symptoms (such as arthralgia, myalgia and fatigue) which commonly occur as extracutaneous manifestations in morphoea. Hydroxychloroquine can also reduce morphoea related skin 'tenderness'.

Ciclosporin

Ciclosporin binds to cyclophilin in the cytosol of lymphocytes, especially T-cells, to inhibit calcineurin induced dephosphorylation of 'nuclear factor of activated T-cells' (NFATc). In turn, this decreases the function of effector T-cells and their release of IL-2 and other related cytokines involved in sclerosis.

In SSc, ciclosporin decreases MMP-9 and may assist with skin softening. Although limited, the efficacy of ciclosporin is reported in a single case of childhood linear morphoea and 6 adults with eosinophilic fasciitis.

FUTURE PERSPECTIVES

As we begin to unravel the complex immunopathology of morphoea and related determinants of disease subsets, precise targets for future treatments are emerging. These include innate responses, specific adaptive response such as B-cell related autoimmunity, Th1 cytokines or Th17 pathways, and/or profibrotic connective tissue repair and developmental signalling pathways (see **Table 2.2**) [6,12,31].

Novel reported therapies and potential future targets

Inflammatory and profibrotic cytokines

A cytokine profile-based conceptual model of the immunopathology of morphoea was recently proposed [32], and has been supported by further cytokine expression profiling. An early (12–24 months) active disease phase characterised by inflammation with a Th1 cytokine response (mediated by IL-2, TNF-α and IL-6) appears to be followed by ongoing inflammation and initiation of fibrosis (>24 months) driven by Th17 related IL-1, IL-17, IL-22 and TGF-β production. Finally, Th2 related IL-4 and IL-13 appear to be linked to the late sclerotic, as well as final atrophic and/or hyperpigmented phases of morphoea morphology [6].

Accordingly, infliximab (chimeric monoclonal antibody to TNF-α) has induced remission in one case of generalised morphoea and three cases of eosinophilic fasciitis. However, etanercept (TNF-α receptor fusion protein) has been linked to the subsequent development of generalised morphoea; whether this was due to injection site related trauma and a subsequent systemic response, or a paradoxical immunological drug response, remains unclear.

IL-6, stimulated by IL-1, is required for wound healing and fibroblast activity, and is intimately involved in morphoea. In response to injury, IL-1, via IL-6 and platelet-derived growth factor (PDGF), promotes fibroblast proliferation, resultant transcription of type I, III and IV collagens and CTGF expression. IL-1 pathways can also activate fibroblasts in SSc. Whilst not yet used in morphoea, tocilizumab (IL-6 receptor monoclonal antibody) has been used with some success in SSc and in five paediatric cases of severe treatment resistant morphoea. In addition, anakinra (IL-1 receptor antagonist) is currently licensed (e.g. in autoinflammatory syndromes) and may have positive effects in morphoea, on a proof of concept basis.

TGF-β is recognized as a potential master regulator of wound healing and a driver of pathological fibrosis [32]. Increased levels of TGF-β and TGF-β receptor-I and II have been demonstrated in skin biopsies and sera of morphoea and SSc patients [32].

Pirfenidone has known antifibrotic effects via TGF-β gene transcription inhibition. Applied topically in a small prospective study of 12 patients with active morphoea, 8% pirfenidone gel demonstrated significant improvements in modified localized scleroderma skin severity index (mLoSSI), durometer induration and histopathological parameters of inflammation and sclerosis after three times daily application for 6 months [33]. Systemically, fresolimumab targets all isoforms of TGF-β and results in significant rapid skin softening in SSc, however, its use may be limited by the evolution of eruptive keratoacanthomas. Guanylate cyclase inhibitors (such as riociguat) also inhibit TGF-β signalling, are approved for use in SSc and ameliorate skin sclerosis in experimental models.

Th17 and T-regulatory cells play a role in sclerosis, and IL-17 appears to be important in morphoea. Low IL-17C with high IL-17E and IL-22 increase fibroblast profibrotic responses which are further enhanced in the presence of IL-22 and TNF activated keratinocytes in both SSc and morphoea. IL-17A also appears important, with levels decreasing in correlation with TGF-β and IL-22 in the setting of polymerised collagen treatment and associated normalisation of dermal architecture in morphoea skin [6].

With brodalimumab (anti-IL-17 receptor-A monoclonal antibody) licensed for use in rheumatoid arthritis, secukinumab and ixekizumab (anti-IL-17A monoclonal antibody) showing excellent results in psoriasis and anti-IL-17E and F antibodies on the horizon, IL-17 as a target in morphoea may have a promising future.

Finally, IL-4 and IL-13 up-regulate collagen synthesis, inhibit collagenase activity and appear to play a role in later phases of morphoea pathogenesis [32]. Dupilumab (IL-4 receptor-α monoclonal antibody) modulates signalling of both IL-4 and IL-13 and could feasibly be of benefit in cases of morphoea who progress rapidly to significant atrophy.

Activated T-cells

Abatacept [recombinant IgG1 fusion protein to cytotoxic T-lymphocyte antigen 4 (CTLA4)] has resulted in significant improvement in two cases of deep and extensive morphoea and further cases of SSc [6].

Antithymocyte globulin (horse or rabbit-derived antibodies against human T-cells, used to prevent and treat GvHD) has been reported in one case of pansclerotic morphoea.

B-cells and autoantibodies

The role of B-cells in morphoea is well recognised. B-cells are known to produce profibrotic cytokines such as IL-6 and TGF-β, promote a profibrotic Th2 response and regulatory B-cells (which inhibit Th1 and Th17) are decreased in SSc [6]. Its autoimmune aetiology is supported by the presence of a variety of autoantibodies [5] and increased serum levels of B-cell activating factor.

Accordingly, intravenous immunoglobulin (IVIg) appears to be effective for skin sclerosis, as well as other organ manifestations of SSc. Hence, there is some rationale for using IVIg in morphoea. To date however, evidence is limited to one single case report of pansclerotic morphoea of childhood, which showed continued improvement with monthly treatments for one year.

Rituximab (anti-CD20 monoclonal antibody) has improved skin and lung fibrosis in SSc, however there are as yet no reports of B-cell depletion therapy in morphoea.

Additional profibrotic pathways and mechanisms in skin fibrosis

Future novel therapeutic targets include a variety of growth factors and signalling pathways known to promote fibrosis, and which may be involved in the immunopathogenesis of morphoea (see **Table 2.2**) [6,31].

Epidermal-dermal morphogenic signalling pathway, Wingless and int homolog (Wnt), is of increasing interest in skin sclerosis, is implicated in SSc and is also of potential relevance to the patterning and morphologic variation seen clinically in morphoea. Wnt-β-catenin signalling and TGF-β pathways are known to interact, and peroxisome proliferator-activated receptor (PPAR)-γ, a recognised antifibrotic receptor which inhibits Wnt-β-catenin signalling, is decreased in SSc, thus promoting fibrosis. Hence, in experimental SSc mouse models, PPAR (γ and α) agonist IVA337 can decrease extracellular matrix deposition and TGF-β related Smad-signalling, and Wnt5a knockout mice appear resistant to bleomycin-induced skin sclerosis.

Of relevance, Fli-1 is a negative regulator of fibrosis, demonstrated to have substantially reduced expression in SSc. Fli-1 knockout mice develop spontaneous skin, lung and oesophageal fibrosis with associated increased levels of IL1, IL6 and IL18. In addition, PDGF is elevated in sclerotic skin lesions and increases SSc fibroblast responsiveness to TGF-β. Although limited by its side effect profile, imatinib (tyrosine kinase inhibitor), via anti-TGF-β, PDGF and Fli-1, prevents fibrogenesis and has shown promising results in three cases of morphoea.

Alpha-melanocyte-stimulating hormone (α-MSH) mediates melanocyte pigment production via melanocortin-1 receptor (MC1R), is up regulated in the epidermis and fibroblasts of human burn wounds and hypertrophic scars, and modulates pro- and anti-inflammatory cytokines produced by keratinocytes, monocytes and fibroblasts. Conversely, and signifying its physiological homeostatic role, α-MSH (via MC1R) antagonises cutaneous fibrosis induced by repeated TGF-β exposure and bleomycin. As such, MC1R

Table 2.2 Potential future treatment targets in morphoea

THERAPY	TARGET	BIOLOGY
Fresolimumab (monoclonal antibody) **Pirfenidone gel** **Pyridone** (derivative, transcription inhibitor)	TGF-β	TGF-β • Is a potential master regulator of pathological fibrosis • Levels are increased in skin and serum of patients with morphoea • Up-regulates MMPs; e.g. MMP12 is over-expressed in SSc
Anakinra (receptor antagonist) **Rilonacept** (receptor fusion protein) **Canakinumab** (antagonist)	IL-1 IL-1 IL-1β	IL-1 • Levels are increased in early to intermediate phase inflammatory/sclerotic morphoea • Promotes fibroblast proliferation, collagen production and CTGF expression • Levels correlate with skin scores
Tocilizumab (monoclonal antibody)	IL-6	Increased levels are seen in early (<24 months) morphoea and correlate with skin scores IL-6, stimulated by IL-1: • Is required for wound healing and fibroblast activity • Promotes fibroblast proliferation and resultant transcription of type I, III and IV collagens and CTGF expression in response to injury • Can activate fibroblasts in SSc • Is intimately involved in morphoea
Secukinumab / Ixekizumab (anti-IL-17A) **Brodalumab** (anti-IL-17 receptor A) **IL-17E or F antibodies**	IL-17	• IL-17 levels are increased in later phase morphoea (24–48 months) • Low IL-17C, with high IL-17E and IL-22 increase fibroblast pro-fibrotic responses • IL-17A levels decrease in correlation with TGF-β and IL-22 in the setting of polymerised collagen treatment
Dupilumab (IL-4 receptor monoclonal antibody)	IL-4 / IL-13	• IL-4/IL-13 up-regulate collagen synthesis and inhibit collagenase activity • IL-4 levels correlate with early inflammatory phase cytokines and skin scores • Increased IL-13 levels correlate with morphoea disease activity
Infliximab (monoclonal antibody) **Etanercept** (fusion protein)	TNF-α	TNF-α • Levels are increased in early phase (<24 months) morphoea • Levels correlate with skin scores
Lisofylline (blocks IL-12 signalling and STAT4 activation)	STAT4	STAT4 • Increases proinflammatory and profibrotic cytokines; eg. TNF-α, IL-2 and IL-6 • Decreases Type-1 IFNs, leading to increased fibrosis
Afamelanotide (αMSH analogue)	αMSH	Homeostatic pathway which modulates pro and anti-inflammatory cytokines to antagonize TGF-β induced skin fibrosis.
Fli-1 (agonist / activation)	Fli-1	Transcription factor; down-regulation induces SSc-like phenotype and enhances skin fibrosis via IL-1, IL-6 and IL-8 over-expression.
IVA337 (agonist)	PPAR (γ and α)	PPAR is involved in: • Promoting fibroblast proliferation, myofibroblast differentiation, collagen and ECM expression • Enhancing epidermal responsiveness to FGF-receptors • Stimulating cytokine production and signalling involved in morphoea related fibrosis; e.g. TNF-α, TGF-β, CTGF, FGF2, Wnt, Shh and Jagged-notched
Imatinib **Bosutinib** (inhibitors)	Tyrosine-kinase	Tyrosine-kinase promotes fibrogenesis via TGF-β, PDGF and Fli-1

knockout mice have demonstrated a susceptibility to fibrosis. It is easy to imagine how these pathways may be linked to the often mixed morphology of sclerosis, atrophy and hyperpigmetation in morphoea, and afamelanotide (synthetic α-MSH) could have a treatment role in some morphoea subsets.

PDE4 inhibition (Apremilast) inhibits fibrosis in a mouse model of sclerotic skin disease, with amelioration of skin sclerosis in sclerodermoid GvHD.

Serotonin/5-hydroxytryptamine (5HT) receptors are elevated in SSc associated interstitial lung disease (ILD) and 5HT stimulation of fibroblasts results in increased collagen production. Promisingly, readily available 5HT-2 blockers, terguride and cyproheptadine, attenuate fibrosis in the bleomycin mouse model and this may be a simple future therapeutic target in morphoea.

Finally, one can also appreciate some therapeutic rationale for autologous haematopoietic stem cell transplantation, which has been useful in SSc [31] and reported in one paediatric case of severe mixed linear and generalised morphoea.

CONCLUSION

Treatment decisions in morphoea must be clinically guided by disease severity assessments which reflect subtype, depth, activity, potential for damage and impact on QoL. Current treatment approaches are largely untargeted. However, as our understanding of the immunopathogenesis of morphoea increases and we begin to unravel the determinants of its heterogeneity, targeted therapies are on the horizon. With this comes the very real possibility of changing outcomes in this potentially debilitating group of conditions.

Key points for clinical practice

- Morphoea is a potentially debilitating condition, and prompt commencement of appropriate therapy can improve patient outcomes.

- Morphoea treatment decisions must be guided by disease severity, which in turn reflects disease subtype (determined using a 3-tiered approach; anatomical distribution, morphology, depth of tissue involvement), level of disease activity, degree of potential irreversible damage and patient focused QoL indices.

- First line treatments include:

  - Topical therapies +/– phototherapy (preferably UVA1 or PUVA) for mild morphoea (limited and superficial)

  - Topical therapies and phototherapy (preferably UVA1 or PUVA) for moderate severity morphoea [superficial generalised (e.g. isomorphic) or superficial linear morphoea of the trunk or limbs (adult onset)]

  - Methotrexate (for at least 2–4 years) and systemic corticosteroids for severe morphoea (linear morphoea (e.g. craniofacial, crossing joints, paediatric onset), generalised morphoea (especially pansclerotic or deep disseminated plaque) and any disease subtype with deep tissue involvement).

- As we unravel the immunopathology underlying the clinical heterogeneity of morphoea, future targeted therapies hold much promise. Anti-IL6 and anti-CTLA4 have shown early positive results in selected cases, and many future targets are evolving.

REFERENCES

1. Li SC, Torok KS, Pope E, et al. Development of consensus treatment plans for juvenile localized scleroderma: a roadmap toward comparative effectiveness studies in juvenile localized scleroderma. Arthritis Care Res 2012; 64:1175–1185.
2. Zwischenberger BA, Jacobe HT. A systematic review of morphea treatments and therapeutic algorithm. J Am Acad Dermatol 2011; 65:925–941.
3. Fett N. Scleroderma: nomenclature, etiology, pathogenesis, prognosis, and treatments: facts and controversies. Clin Dermatol 2013; 31:432–437.
4. Fett N, Werth VP. Update on morphea: part I. Epidemiology, clinical presentation, and pathogenesis. J Am Acad Dermatol 2011; 64:217–228.
5. Pequet MS, Holland KE, Zhao S, et al. Risk factors for morphoea disease severity: a retrospective review of 114 paediatric patients. Br J Dermatol 2014; 170:895–900.
6. Saracino AM, Denton CP, Orteu CH. The molecular pathogenesis of morphoea: from genetics to future treatment targets. Br J Dermatol 2017; 177:34–46.
7. Zulian F, Cuffaro G, Sperotto F. Scleroderma in children: an update. Current Opin Rheumatol 2013; 25:643–650.
8. Fett N, Werth VP. Update on morphea: part II. Outcome measures and treatment. J Am Acad Dermatol 2011; 64:231–242.
9. Kelsey CE, Torok KS. The Localized Scleroderma Cutaneous Assessment Tool: responsiveness to change in a pediatric clinical population. J Am Acad Dermatol 2013; 69:214–220.
10. Das S, Bernstein I, Jacobe H. Correlates of self-reported quality of life in adults and children with morphea. J Am Acad Dermatol 2014; 70:904–910.
11. Kim A, Marinkovich N, Vasquez R, et al. Clinical features of patients with morphea and the pansclerotic subtype: a cross-sectional study from the morphea in adults and children cohort. J Rheumatol 2014; 41:106–112.
12. Distler O, Cozzio A. Systemic sclerosis and localized scleroderma--current concepts and novel targets for therapy. Semin Immunopathol 2016; 38:87–95.
13. Nouri S, Jacobe H. Recent developments in diagnosis and assessment of morphea. Curr Rheumatol Rep 2013; 15:308.
14. Warburton KL, McPhee MJ, Savage LJ, et al. Management of morphoea: results of a national survey of UK clinicians. Br J Dermatol 2014; 171:1243–1245.
15. Gordon Spratt EA, Gorcey LV, Soter NA, et al. Phototherapy, photodynamic therapy and photophoresis in the treatment of connective-tissue diseases: a review. Br J Dermatol 2015; 173:19–30.
16. Pavlotsky F, Sakka N, Lozinski A, et al. Bath psoralen-UVA photochemotherapy for localized scleroderma: experience from a single institute. Photodermatol Photoimmunol Photomed 2013; 29:247–252.
17. Pileri A, Raone B, Raboni R, et al. Generalized morphea successfully treated with extracorporeal photochemotherapy (ECP). Dermatol Online J 2014; 20:21258.
18. Nistico SP, Saraceno R, Schipani C, et al. Different applications of monochromatic excimer light in skin diseases. Photomed Laser Surg 2009; 27:647–654.
19. Zulian F, Martini G, Vallongo C, et al. Methotrexate treatment in juvenile localized scleroderma: a randomized, double-blind, placebo-controlled trial. Arthritis Rheum 2011; 63:1998–2006.
20. Schanz S, Henes J, Ulmer A, et al. Response evaluation of musculoskeletal involvement in patients with deep morphea treated with methotrexate and prednisolone: a combined MRI and clinical approach. Am J Roentgenol 2013; 200:W376–382.
21. Lebeaux D, Frances C, Barete S, et al. Eosinophilic fasciitis (Shulman disease): new insights into the therapeutic management from a series of 34 patients. Rheumatology (Oxford, England) 2012; 51:557–561.
22. Berianu F, Cohen MD, Abril A, et al. Eosinophilic fasciitis: clinical characteristics and response to methotrexate. Int J Rheum Dis 2015; 18:91–98.
23. Torok KS, Arkachaisri T. Methotrexate and corticosteroids in the treatment of localized scleroderma: a standardized prospective longitudinal single-center study. J Rheumatol 2012; 39:286–294.
24. Koch SB, Cerci FB, Jorizzo JL, et al. Linear morphea: a case series with long-term follow-up of young, methotrexate-treated patients. J Dermatol Treat 2013; 24:435–438.
25. Mirsky L, Chakkittakandiyil A, Laxer RM, et al. Relapse after systemic treatment in paediatric morphoea. Br J Dermatol 2012; 166:443–445.
26. Zulian F, Vallongo C, Patrizi A, et al. A long-term follow-up study of methotrexate in juvenile localized scleroderma (morphea). J Am Acad Dermatol 2012; 67:1151–1156.
27. Mertens JS, Seyger MM, Kievit W, et al. Disease recurrence in localized scleroderma: a retrospective analysis of 344 patients with paediatric- or adult-onset disease. Br J Dermatol 2015; 172:722–728.

28. Zhang G, Xu T, Zhang H, et al. [Randomized control multi-center clinical study of mycophenolate mofetil and cyclophosphamide in the treatment of connective tissue disease related interstitial lung disease]. Zhonghua Yi Xue Za Zhi 2015; 95:3641–3645.
29. Omair MA, Alahmadi A, Johnson SR. Safety and effectiveness of mycophenolate in systemic sclerosis. A systematic review. PloS One 2015; 10:e0124205.
30. Hinchcliff M, Huang CC, Wood TA, et al. Molecular signatures in skin associated with clinical improvement during mycophenolate treatment in systemic sclerosis. J Invest Dermatol 2013; 133:1979–1989.
31. Ciechomska M, van Laar J, O'Reilly S. Current frontiers in systemic sclerosis pathogenesis. Exp Dermatol 2015; 24:401–406.
32. Kurzinski K, Torok KS. Cytokine profiles in localized scleroderma and relationship to clinical features. Cytokine 2011; 55:157–164.
33. Rodriguez-Castellanos M, Tlacuilo-Parra A, Sanchez-Enriquez S, et al. Pirfenidone gel in patients with localized scleroderma: a phase II study. Arthritis Res Ther 2014; 16:510.

Chapter 3

Update on the management of chronic urticaria

Nadine Marrouche, Clive Grattan

INTRODUCTION

Chronic urticaria (CU) is a disease characterised by the development of itchy weals, angioedema, or both for more than 6 weeks. It is mediated by mast cell degranulation, which can be immunological or nonimmunological, leading to release of proinflammatory mediators including histamine [1]. It comprises several subtypes which are classified according to clinical pattern rather than etiology. The latter remains poorly understood in general despite abundant literature on the role of functional autoantibodies in the pathogenesis of the disease in more than a third of patients. The disease can cause significant disability affecting an individual's quality of life (QoL) and has a high economic burden with considerable health care costs [1]. Antihistamines have long been the mainstay, and at standard dose, the only licensed treatment for CU until the advent of omalizumab. This has encouraged a new interest in CU, not only because of its efficacy but also as it shed new insights into the pathophysiology of the disease and increased interest in research in the field. There is a sizable medical literature on the treatment of various subtypes of urticaria. This chapter will only cover current evidence-based management of the disease.

DISEASE TERMINOLOGY AND CLASSIFICATION

Chronic urticaria is divided into two main types. Chronic spontaneous urticaria (CSU) is characterised by the spontaneous appearance of weals and/or angioedema lasting for 24–48 hours. It is a relatively common disease with a point prevalence of 0.5–1% and a female predominance [2]. The inducible urticaria subtypes are each triggered by a specific and reproducible stimulus and resolve in less than 2 hours with the exception of delayed pressure urticaria. It is not uncommon for CSU and chronic inducible urticaria to overlap in some patients (**Figure 3.1**). Although the terms CSU and chronic idiopathic urticaria (CIU) are still used interchangeably in the medical literature, there has been an emphasis

Nadine Marrouche MD, Consultant Dermatologist, Dermatology Department, Norfolk and Norwich University Hospitals NHS Foundation Trust, Norwich, UK

Clive Grattan MA, MD, FRCP, Consultant Dermatologist, St John's Institute of Dermatology, Guy's Hospital, London, UK. Email: Clive.E.Grattan@gsst.nhs.uk (for correspondence)

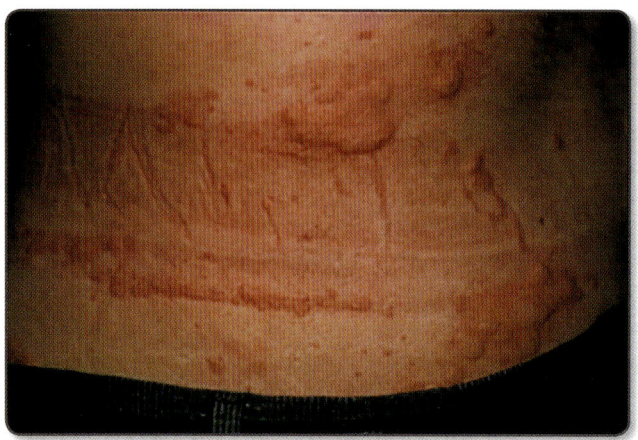

Figure 3.1 Chronic spontaneous urticaria and delayed pressure urticaria overlap.

in the latest urticaria consensus meeting on adopting the term CSU to refer to the disease [3]. CSU encompasses both chronic idiopathic and chronic autoimmune urticarias. Chronic inducible urticaria is further divided into subtypes, each a disease entity on its own (**Table 3.1**). It is important to differentiate urticaria from other medical conditions where weals, angioedema, or both can occur as a symptom like the autoinflammatory syndromes and from diseases that have been associated with urticaria for historical reasons like maculopapular cutaneous mastocytosis (urticaria pigmentosa) [1].

CHRONIC URTICARIA DIAGNOSIS AND ASSESSMENT TOOLS

The diagnosis of CSU is mostly based on a good medical history. Skin examination can be normal on clinical presentation due to the recurring nature of the disease. Unless suggested otherwise by the history and/or physical examination, no specific laboratory investigations are needed in the evaluation of CSU, as it is unlikely to identify an underlying etiology. Some clinicians measure the level of thyroid autoantibodies to identify circumstantial evidence for autoimmunity as an underlying cause for CSU. In addition, their presence could indicate a poorer disease prognosis with a longer course and more severe symptoms [4]. The diagnosis of an inducible urticaria is also based on a detailed medical history but should always be confirmed by a challenge test that aims to induce the rash by reproducing the stimulus that triggers it. The test should also help determine trigger thresholds, which provide objective measures for assessing disease severity and response to treatment [1].

Objective assessment tools have been developed to assess disease severity and its impact on QoL. These are also important to monitor patients while on treatment. The dermatology life quality index (DLQI) questionnaire is still widely used to measure the impact of the disease on patients' QoL although a disease-specific tool known as chronic urticaria quality of life questionnaire (CU-Q2oL) has proven to be superior and more sensitive [5]. As for disease severity, the urticaria activity score (UAS) is now a validated test that combines the daily number of weals and pruritus severity scores to create a daily score ranging from 0 to 6. The sum of UAS scores over 7 consecutive days (UAS7) has been used as an endpoint in many trials assessing the efficacy of omalizumab in CSU and is

Table 3.1. Current classification of chronic urticaria	
Chronic spontaneous urticaria	**Chronic inducible urticaria (known trigger)**
No known eliciting factor	Symptomatic dermographism (mechanical shearing pressure)
	Delayed pressure urticaria (vertical pressure)
	Solar urticaria (ultraviolet and/or visible light)
	Heat urticaria (localised heat contact)
	Cold urticaria (cold contact)
	Vibratory angioedema (vibratory force)
	Cholinergic urticaria (change in core body temperature)
	Contact urticaria (contact with causal substance)
	Aquagenic urticaria (water contact)

now commonly used in clinical practice[5]. More recently, a new tool, the angioedema activity score (AAS), has been developed to assess disease activity in patients with recurrent angioedema, which is not assessed by the UAS [6].

CHRONIC URTICARIA TREATMENT

The management of CU is mostly pharmacological and aims at controlling the symptoms of the disease including pruritus as well as improving the QoL. In CSU, certain lifestyle modifications like heat and alcohol avoidance can be beneficial in some patients but mostly when combined with medical treatment. Avoiding the culprit trigger can alleviate an inducible urticaria but this is often a practical challenge. The most recent European guidelines for the management of urticaria have focused on evidence-based treatment options. These include H1-antihistamines as a mainstay therapy, to be supplemented with ciclosporin, omalizumab, or montelukast in case of antihistamine failure. Medications like H2-antihistamines, dapsone, and methotrexate, although still widely used in clinical practice, are no longer endorsed by these guidelines due to lack of trial evidence. Most of these therapies appear to work in CU by mechanisms that are yet to be elucidated. It is recommended to monitor the disease response to any of the above therapies by using the objective assessment tools and to stop the treatment when symptoms have settled to establish whether the disease has gone into spontaneous remission. Treatment can be restarted when the condition relapses. Indeed, it is reported that 80% of CSU patients become symptom-free after just 1 year of disease activity [2].

ANTIHISTAMINES

Antihistamines have been used in the treatment of urticaria since the 1950s and remain the mainstay of treatment. There is a long-standing experience among medical practitioners in the use of sedating H1-antihistamines but concern about their safety emerged over the past few decades in relation to sedation, especially with updosing. Most current guidelines recommend against their use [7]. Nonsedating H1-antihistamines (2nd generation) are first-line treatment for CU. They have all been shown to be effective in controlling the symptoms of urticaria but none stands out as the most effective [8]. For years, they have been, at the standard dose, the only licensed treatment for CU, until omalizumab was licensed in 2014 as well. Studies have shown they are often significantly more effective at higher doses in both the spontaneous and inducible types of CU. The current European guidelines propose up-dosing H1-antihistamines up to 4 times the licensed dose, if necessary, before considering other treatment options, and there is real world evidence to show this practice is safe. Most studies have evaluated the updosing of a single antihistamine and hence the guidelines recommend this approach over combining different H1-antihistamines. However, studies have shown that up to one-third of patients show resistance to antihistamine therapy [9].

OMALIZUMAB

Omalizumab is a humanised anti-IgE monoclonal antibody. It has been intensively studied in the field of allergic asthma for which it is a licensed treatment. Although the specific mechanism of action of omalizumab in CU is still unknown, it is thought to increase mast cell stability by sequestering free IgE and subsequently down-regulating membrane bound FcεRI [10]. Several multicentre randomised controlled trials have demonstrated the efficacy and safety of omalizumab in CSU irrespective of autoimmune status and background therapy for the disease. Overall, the use of omalizumab at a dose of 300 mg demonstrated the best results in controlling CSU symptoms and improving QoL [11–14]. Omalizumab appears to be effective not only in reducing pruritus and number of weals but also in alleviating angioedema when it is a component of CSU [15,16]. It is the only licensed treatment for H1-antihistamine resistant CSU patients. A real-world retrospective study of CSU patient cohorts treated with omalizumab and ciclosporin showed better outcomes and improved QoL with omalizumab [17]. The practice of prescribing omalizumab is different among various centres in the world. In the UK, the National Institute for Health and Care Excellence (NICE) recommends omalizumab as an add-on therapy for treating severe CSU in adults and young people aged 12 years and above. Patients should demonstrate inadequate response to H1-antihistamines with montelukast (UAS7 scores ≥28) to be eligible for therapy. Omalizumab is administered as a 300-mg subcutaneous injection every 4 weeks for a total of 6 months. According to NICE guidance, omalizumab should be stopped before or at the fourth dose if CSU has not responded to treatment. At the end of a 6 months treatment cycle, omalizumab is also stopped to re-assess disease activity and can be restarted if the disease relapses. Patients should be monitored for signs of anaphylaxis following each injection although no confirmed cases have been reported in CSU patients to date. Therapy is monitored using objective disease assessment tools (UAS7 and DLQI) and there is no need for baseline or monitoring biochemical tests [18]. More studies are needed to establish the mechanism of action and optimum treatment duration of omalizumab in CSU. Although not licensed for inducible urticaria, there are several case reports/series on efficacy of omalizumab in various subtypes of inducible urticaria [19,20]. Omalizumab has been observed to be effective and safe in children as young as 2 and in pregnant woman but the data is based on individual case reports/series and its use in such settings is only recommended when the expected benefit outweighs any potential risk [20–22].

CICLOSPORIN

Ciclosporin is so far the best-studied immune modulator in the treatment of CSU. There is strong evidence-based data to support its efficacy, in daily doses ranging between 3–5 mg/kg, in the treatment of recalcitrant disease, usually as add on-therapy to H1-antihistamines [23,24]. Its long-term use is limited by its potentially serious side effects including increased serum creatinine and hypertension. Patients should be closely monitored accordingly. Most of these effects are dose-related and reversible on discontinuation of therapy and it appears that a lower dose of the drug (2–3 mg/kg/day) is better tolerated while still effective in CSU. In addition, long-term use of ciclosporin in transplant recipients has been associated with an increased risk of malignancy [25]. Ciclosporin has been shown to be more effective in patients with positive basophil histamine release assay, which is used as a marker for autoimmune urticarial [26]. In general however, phenotyping patients is not required before treatment.

MONTELUKAST

Montelukast is a leukotriene receptor antagonist. In the UK, it is licensed in the prophylactic treatment of asthma and to relieve symptoms of seasonal allergic rhinitis in patients with asthma. There is evidence to support its added therapeutic benefit in the treatment of CSU when used in combination with H1-antihistamines but not when used as monotherapy [27]. A therapeutic response is usually expected in the first 3 weeks of treatment beyond which therapy should be discontinued if the disease remains symptomatic [28]. It is recommended as add-on therapy if antihistamine monotherapy fails in the US guidelines whereas the European guidelines advocate its use only when up-dosing antihistamines has failed. There are anecdotal reports about its efficacy, along with H1-antistamines, in the treatment of some types of inducible urticaria with most evidence for delayed pressure urticaria [29].

ORAL CORTICOSTEROIDS

The efficacy of systemic corticosteroids in the treatment of different types of CU is well established and they are included in CU treatment algorithms of international guidelines. However, there is only one retrospective study on their use in CU, which might explain why there is no widely agreed therapeutic regime of their use to treat the disease [30]. The current European guidelines recommend a short course (maximum of 10 days) of oral corticosteroids to control acute flares of CU despite treatment with first, second, or third line agents. As such, corticosteroids continue to play an important role in the management of CU but are regarded a rescue rather than mainstay treatment.

FUTURE PERSPECTIVES

There have been important changes in the management of CU over the last decade. There is general agreement among CU experts to use a more specific terminology and to simplify the classification of the disease. New disease assessment tools are now widely used. These not only provide an objective way of assessing disease severity but also emphasize the importance of considering the disease' significant impact on QoL. The most recent guidelines have focused on simple stepwise therapeutic algorithms with evidence-based and safer treatment options. However, there remain unmet needs in the management of CU. Real-world data has demonstrated heterogeneity in patients' response to various treatments implying different phenotypes for the disease. This is still poorly understood and more evidence is required to shed light on this observation and eventually help us better understand the pathophysiology of the disease. It has been suggested that identification of potential biomarkers to monitor CSU activity and response to treatment would help clinicians predict disease outcomes and propose more specific treatment algorithms [31].

Key points for clinical practice

- Chronic spontaneous urticaria (CSU) is the most common type of chronic urticaria.
- Although the pathophysiology of CSU remains poorly understood, there have been major advances in the management of the disease over the past few years.
- Omalizumab is now licensed for the treatment of CSU and appears to be a more effective and safer treatment than immunosuppressive therapies.

REFERENCES

1. Zuberbier T, Aberer W, Asero R, et al. The EAACI/ GA^{2}LEN /EDF/WAO Guideline for the definition, classification, diagnosis, and management of urticaria: the 2013 revision and update. Allergy 2014; 69:868–887.
2. Maurer M, Weller K, Bindslev-Jensen C, et al. Unmet clinical needs in chronic spontaneous urticaria. A GA^{2}LEN task force report. Allergy 2011; 66:317–330.
3. Maurer M, Bindslev-Jensen C, Giménez-Arnau A, et al. Chronic idiopathic urticaria (CIU) is no longer idiopathic: time for an update. Br J Dermatol 2013; 168:455–456.
4. Lee SY, Song WJ, Jung JW, et al. Thyroid autoantibodies and the prognosis of chronic idiopathic urticaria. Allergy Asthma Respir Dis 2013; 1:151–156.
5. Baiardini I, Braido F, Bindslev-Jensen C, et al. Recommendations for assessing patient-reported outcomes and health-related quality of life in patients with urticaria: a GA^{2}LEN taskforce position paper. Allergy 2011; 66:840–844.
6. Weller K, Groffik A, Magerl M, et al. Development, validation, and initial results of the Angioedema Activity Score. Allergy 2013; 68:1185–1192.
7. Staevska M, Gugutkova M, Lazarova C, et al. Night-time sedating H1-antihistamine increases daytime somnolence but not treatment efficacy in chronic spontaneous urticaria: a randomized controlled trial. Br J Dermatol 2014; 171:148–154.
8. Sharma M, Bennett C, Cohen SN, Carter B. H1-antihistamines for chronic spontaneous urticaria. Cochrane Database Syst Rev 2014; 14:CD006137.
9. Weller K, Viehmann K, Bräutigam M, et al. Management of chronic spontaneous urticaria in real life – in accordance with the guidelines? A cross-sectional physician-based survey study. J Eur Acad Dermatol Venereol 2013; 27:43–50.
10. Zuberbier T, Maurer M. Omalizumab for the treatment of chronic urticaria. Expert Rev Clin Immunol 2015; 11:171–180.
11. Maurer M, Rosén K, Hsieh HJ, et al. Omalizumab for the treatment of chronic idiopathic or spontaneous urticaria. N Engl J Med 2013; 368:924–935.
12. Kaplan A, Ledford D, Ashby M, et al. Omalizumab in patients with symptomatic chronic idiopathic/ spontaneous urticaria despite standard combination therapy. J Allergy Clin Immunol 2013; 132:101–109.
13. Saini SS, Bindslev-Jensen C, Maurer M, et al. Efficacy and safety of omalizumab in patients with chronic idiopathic/spontaneous urticaria who remain symptomatic on H1 antihistamines: a randomized placebo-controlled study. J Invest Dermatol 2015; 135:67–75.
14. Casale TB, Bernstein JA, Maurer M, et al. Similar efficacy with omalizumab in chronic idiopathic/ spontaneous urticaria despite different background therapy. J Allergy Clin Immunol Pract 2015; 3:743–750.
15. Zazzali JL, Kaplan A, Maurer M, et al. Angioedema in the omalizumab chronic idiopathic/spontaneous urticaria pivotal studies. Ann Allergy Asthma Immunol 2016; 117:370–377e1.
16. Staubach P, Metz M, Chapman-Rothe N, et al. Effect of omalizumab on angioedema in H1-antihistamine-resistant chronic spontaneous urticaria patients: results from X-ACT, a randomized controlled trial. Allergy 2016; 71:1135–1144.

17. Savic S, Marsland A, McKay D, et al. Retrospective case note review of chronic spontaneous urticaria outcomes and adverse effects in patients treated with omalizumab or ciclosporin in UK secondary care. Allergy Asthma Clin Immunol 2015; 11:21.

18. National Institute of Health and Care Excellence (NICE). NICE technology appraisal guidance 339: Omalizumab for previously treated chronic spontaneous urticarial, June 2015.

19. Müller S, Rafei-Shamsabadi D, Technau-Hafsi K, Renzel S, Jakob T. Bullous Delayed Pressure Urticaria Responding to Omalizumab. Acta Derm Venereol 2016; 96:416–417.

20. Alba Marín JC, Martorell Aragones A, et al. Treatment of Severe Cold-Induced Urticaria in a Child With Omalizumab. J Investig Allergol Clin Immunol 2015; 25:303–304.

21. Ghazanfar MN, Thomsen SF. Successful and Safe Treatment of Chronic Spontaneous Urticaria with Omalizumab in a Woman during Two Consecutive Pregnancies. Case Rep Med 2015; 2015:368053.

22. Cuervo-Pardo L, Barcena-Blanch M, Radojicic C. Omalizumab use during pregnancy for CIU: a tertiary care experience. Eur Ann Allergy Clin Immunol 2016; 48:145–146.

23. Grattan CE, O'Donnell BF, Francis DM, et al. Randomized double-blind study of cyclosporin in chronic 'idiopathic' urticaria. Br J Dermatol 2000; 143:365–372.

24. Vena GA, Cassano N, Colombo D, Peruzzi E, Pigatto P; Neo-I-30 Study Group. Cyclosporine in chronic idiopathic urticaria: a double-blind, randomized, placebo-controlled trial. J Am Acad Dermatol 2006; 55:705–709.

25. Kessel A, Toubi E. Cyclosporine-A in severe chronic urticaria: the option for long-term therapy. Allergy 2010; 65:1478–1482.

26. Iqbal K, Bhargava K, Skov PS, Falkencrone S, Grattan CE. A positive serum basophil histamine release assay is a marker for ciclosporin-responsiveness in patients with chronic spontaneous urticaria. Clin Transl Allergy 2012; 2:19.

27. de Silva NL, Damayanthi H, Rajapakse AC, Rodrigo C, Rajapakse S. Leukotriene receptor antagonists in monotherapy or in combination with antihistamines in the treatment of chronic urticaria: a systematic review. Allergy Asthma Clin Immunol 2014; 10:24.

28. Greenberger PA. Chronic urticaria: new management options. World Allergy Organ J 2014; 7:31.

29. Nettis E, Colanardi MC, Soccio AL, Ferrannini A, Vacca A. Desloratadine in combination with montelukast suppresses the dermographometer challenge test papule, and is effective in the treatment of delayed pressure urticaria: a randomized, double-blind, placebo-controlled study. Br J Dermatol 2006; 155:1279–1282.

30. Asero R, Tedeschi A. Usefulness of a short course of oral prednisone in antihistamine-resistant chronic urticaria: a retrospective analysis. J Investig Allergol Clin Immunol 2010; 20:386–390.

31. Giménez-Arnau AM, Toubi E, Marsland AM, Maurer M. Clinical management of urticaria using omalizumab: the first licensed biological therapy available for chronic spontaneous urticaria. J Eur Acad Dermatol Venereol 2016; 30:25–32.

Chapter 4

New concepts in the management of alopecia areata

Shirin Zaheri, Sarah Hogan, Marie C Wilmot, Iaisha Ali

INTRODUCTION

Background

Alopecia areata (AA) is the most common cause of immune mediated hair loss. It commonly presents as discrete patches of hair loss of the scalp. Other sites can also be affected including the eyelash, eyebrow and beard hair. More extensive loss of scalp hair (known as alopecia totalis) and body (alopecia universalis) can occur.

The disease can occur at any age with peak onset between 20 and 30 years [1], and is the commonest cause of hair loss in children [2]. A recent systematic review by Villasante Fricke and Miteva [1] showed that the lifetime incidence of AA is 2% and may be increasing. Associated comorbidities include Hashimoto's thyroiditis, atopy, psoriasis and diabetes mellitus [1]. Although alopecia is not life-threatening it can be associated with a significant degree of psychosocial stress. AA is associated with depression and anxiety in up to 39% and 62% of patients respectively. Female AA sufferers are more likely to report poor quality of life than males [1].

Evidence for an immunological basis of AA has recently become evident and it is now understood to be a T-cell mediated autoimmune disorder. Patients experience acute alopecia due to loss of hair follicle immune privilege (IP) [3]. Hair loss is induced through interference and arrest of the growth phase of the hair cycle (anagen), leading to premature follicle senescence rather than direct immune-mediated follicle destruction.

The disease process is unpredictable and the natural history variable between patients. Hair follicle miniaturisation renders the follicle unable to re-enter anagen, which initially affects one or many patches and may progress to alopecia totalis or universalis. Factors associated with extensive disease include younger age of onset, positive family history, nail signs, associated autoimmune disease and atopy [1]. The presentation of the condition also affects prognosis, with alopecia ophiasis, totalis and universalis presenting the most challenges.

Shirin Zaheri BSc (Hons) MBBS MRCP PGCME, Consultant Dermatologist & Senior Honorary Lecturer, Charing Cross Hospital, Imperial College Healthcare NHS Trust, London, UK

Sarah Hogan BSc (Hons) MBBS MRCP PGCME, Clinical Fellow, Imperial College Healthcare NHS Trust, London, UK

Marie C Wilmot MRes MBBS MRCP, Dermatology Trainee, AFHEA Imperial College Healthcare NHS Trust, London, UK

Iaisha Ali MB ChB MRCP MSc, Consultant Dermatologist, HCA Harley Street Clinic, London, UK

Since the clinical and histological presentations of AA are distinctive it is not usually a diagnostic challenge, however it is difficult to manage. Treatment options range from topical applications to systemic treatments that aim to reduce inflammation. The physician should also consider the impact on the patient's life and offer support in the form of wigs or counselling when appropriate. Spontaneous remission is possible but mainly seen in those with a short history of small areas of alopecia [4].

Until recently there have been very few randomised controlled trials (RCTs) for AA treatments [5] , as presentations and levels of disease activity amongst patients are so variable making it difficult to control for. Half-head control studies contribute to case series but not until relatively recently were there many placebo-controlled studies [6]. When interpreting any study on AA it is worth noting whether the type of AA has been considered from the outset and whether suitable comparisons have been made (e.g. universalis or totalis, chronic or acute). Spontaneous remission may occur in the less severe variants of AA, which may cloud interpretation [7]. Authors might use a variety of outcome measures such as the severity of alopecia tool (SALT) score [8] or hair growth index. These can be combined with patient assessment using tools such as the visual analogue scale or quality of life questionnaires.

Current options and the need for new management strategies

Topical and intralesional application of very potent steroids have been shown to be effective and can lead to long-term regrowth. However, this is more suitable for smaller patches of alopecia and often patients fail treatment or have variable responses that are possibly related to disease severity [9,10]. Topical steroid application can cause folliculitis, scalp atrophy, telangiectasia, hypopigmentation, discomfort and adrenal suppression, and efficacy of potent steroid application under occlusion is suboptimal [10–12]. Although systemic steroids can also be used, the benefits of long term treatment often do not outweigh the risks [7]. To minimise these risks minipulse therapy can be used and has been shown to be effective, although the uncontrolled year long study that showed this by Khaitan et al. [13] was relatively small with only 16 patients, and disease duration can effect outcomes with pulsed oral steroid therapy [14] .

Another alternative to topical steroid therapy is topical immunotherapy with irritants such as 2,3-diphenylcyclopropenone (DPCP), which have been shown to be effective [14,16], but responses are highly variable and those with more severe disease may be less likely to respond [17]. Side effects of contact immunotherapy include dermatitis, urticaria and vitiligo [7]. Current UK guidelines suggest the use of topical and intralesional steroids in patchy AA, or contact immunotherapy +/– wigs in more widespread disease [7].

There have been reports of successful treatment with Psoralen plus UVA, however, the results of these should be interpreted with caution as these were not controlled studies [18,19]. There are mixed reports regarding the efficacy of topical minoxidil [20–22] and the general consensus is that it is not sufficiently effective, neither is topical Tacrolimus [23] or Anthralin [24,25].

For those favouring alternative measures, a double-blind randomised control trial showed that massage of topical aromatherapy is significantly more effective than massage alone in the treatment of AA, with 44% of the treatment group showing an improvement in investigator-assessed photographic appearance after 7 months treatment compared to 15% in the control group [26]. Importantly, hypnotherapy in patients with AA has been shown to help reduce associated feelings of anxiety or depression [27].

Systemic treatments are usually reserved for more severe cases, and various attempts have been made to identify suitable candidates. Two studies have shown anti-TNF drugs to be unsuccessful treatment options [28,29], and there have been reports of anti-TNF drugs triggering AA [30]. Methotrexate, although not widely used, has been shown to be effective in a non-controlled study of patients with severe long-standing AA, with 14 out of 22 showing some response after a mean follow-up period of 11 years [31]. In this study, concomitant prednisolone administration increased the likelihood of hair regrowth. Subsequent retrospective noncontrolled studies to support this have shown that it is safe and that long-term maintenance treatment is necessary to prevent relapse [32–34]. A phase III trial comparing Methotrexate with placebo for AA is currently underway at the University of Rouen, France [35]. Ciclosporin A (CsA), thought to act by suppressing aberrant T-cell activity, has been shown to be effective at inducing hair regrowth in several noncontrolled studies, with or without adjuvant corticosteroids, with variable response rates [36–40]. However, it has been demonstrated to be less effective (in combination with low-dose oral corticosteroid) than pulsed high-dose oral corticosteroid alone [14], and there have been reports of AA occurring in patients taking CsA for other reasons [41–46]. An attempt has been made at combined therapy with PUVA, although the risk of malignancy is heightened when combining these treatments [44]. Disease duration influences response to CsA treatment, relapse is common and adverse events affect treatment compliance [40,45]; attempts to create effective topical CsA treatments have failed [46–48].

In summary, current treatment options are untargeted and unsatisfactory. The prognosis for severe or long-standing AA is generally poor, and next-generation treatment options are necessary to provide adequate therapeutic options. Moreover, there is evidence to suggest that the disease process shares similarities with other antigen- and organ-specific T-cell mediated diseases such as type 1 diabetes [49], therefore AA research may also contribute to our overall understanding of autoimmune diseases.

IDENTIFYING NEW TREATMENT TARGETS

Healthy follicles: the immune privilege

It is well established that healthy hair is protected from the immune system by IP. IP of hair follicles was discovered when in 1971, Billingham allotransplanted melanocytic epidermis into genetically incompatible guinea pigs [50]. The animal model showed sparing of hair pigmentation despite immune-mediated loss of pigment in the allogenic epidermis (see **Figure 4.1**, taken from Paus et al. 2005) [51]. Paus found that specifically the proximal epithelium of anagen follicles have IP, which keeps follicle autoantigens 'hidden' maintains immune privilege.

Further research has shown that healthy hair is protected from the immune system by a number of intrinsic mechanisms and external features (**Table 4.1**). These include a paucity of immune cells at the follicle and reduced expression of autoantigens via the normal mechanism of MHC-I expression. The follicle is also shielded by protective molecules that act to create a locally immunosuppressed environment.

Loss of the immune privilege in alopecia areata

In patients with AA, the follicle loses its protective mechanisms through T-cell mediated processes. T cell release of IL-15 and IFN-γ causes proliferation of NKG2D+ T cells via Janus

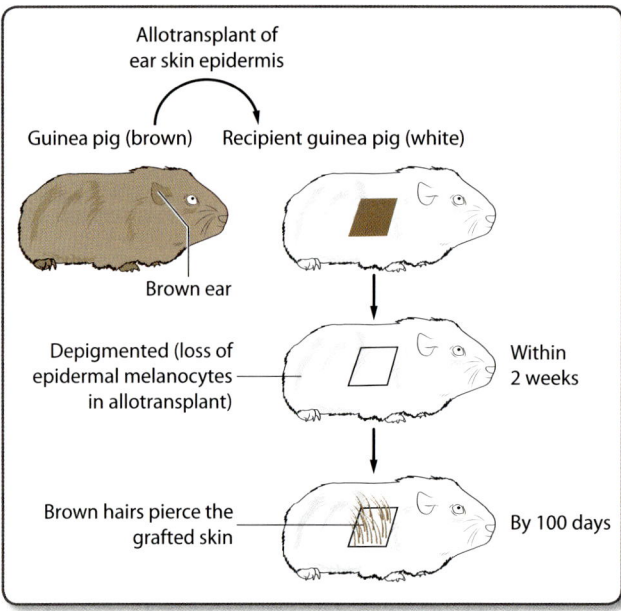

Figure 4.1 The hair follicle IP (taken from Paus et al. 2005) [51]. Epidermis from the pigmented donor is transplanted into the skin of the white host. Within 2 weeks the host rejects the allogenic melanocytes, causing the graft to lose its colour. By 100 days, the graft begins to develop pigmented hairs, indicating that melanocytes within the hair bulbs were protected from the host immune system.

Table 4.1: Mechanisms of hair follicle immune privilege maintenance [51] (adapted from Paus et al. 2005)	
External feature	**Protective mechanism**
Paucity of lymphatics in local epithelium	Physical barrier to all immune cells
Paucity of local Langerhans cells and lack of MHC-II expression (causing functional impairment)	Protection from Langerhans cells
Extracellular matrix production	Physical barrier to immune cells
Intrinsic feature	**Protective mechanism**
Down regulation of classical MHC-I expression in anagen hair bulbs and of melanocytes in the hair follicle	Impaired antigen presentation to autoreactive CD8+ T cells
Downregulation of MHC-I-related molecules, e.g. β2-microglobulin	Impaired antigen-presentation due to instability of any remaining MHC-1
Expression of non-classical MHC-I (MHC-Ib, and HLA-G)	Inhibition of natural killer cells
Expression of Fas ligand	Apoptosis of autoreactive T cells
Expression of protective molecules such as transforming growth factor-β1 (TGF-β1) or TGF-β2, interleukin-10, calcitonin gene-related peptide, α-melanocyte-stimulating hormone and macrophage migration inhibitory factor	Local immunosuppression

kinase signal transducer and activator of transcription (JAK-STAT) pathways. IFN-☒ then upregulates MHC-I, which exposes hair follicle autoantigens that are thought to originate from keratinocytes and melanocytes [52], leading to IP collapse (see **Figure 4.2**).

In addition to JAK-STAT pathway activation, T regulatory cells are implicated in the pathophysiology of AA. When functioning properly these cells have been found to

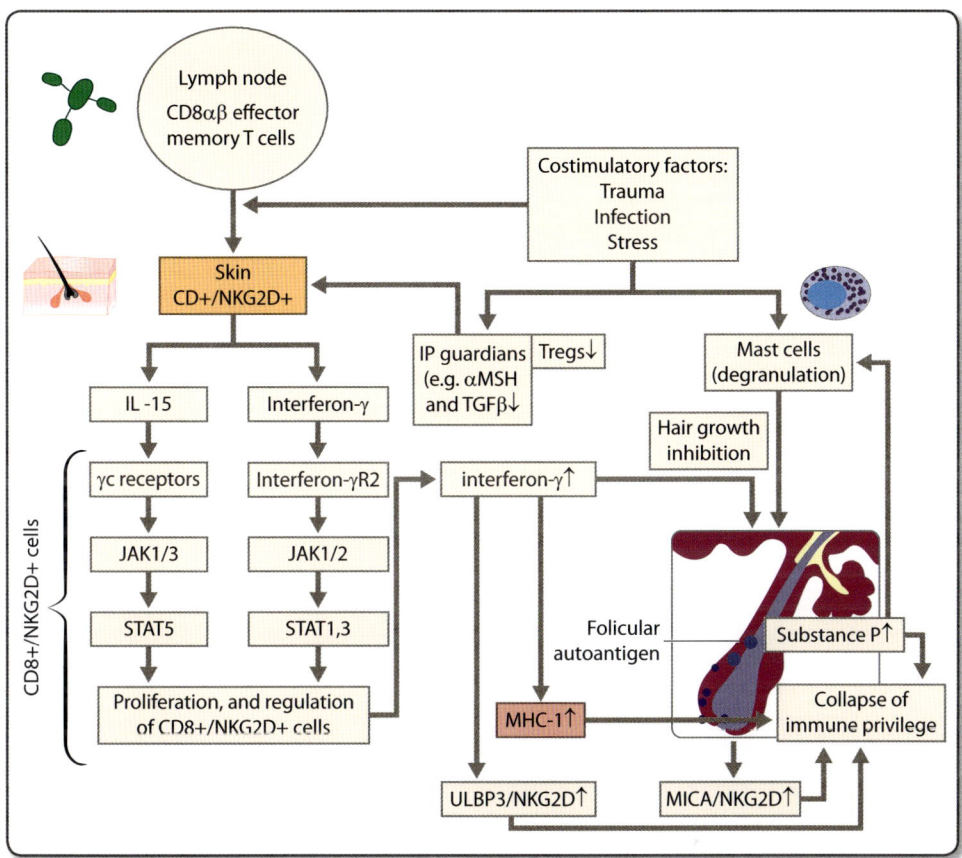

Figure 4.2 The pathogenesis of AA (taken from Gilhar, 2016) [3]. In susceptible individuals, T cells expressing NKG2D release IFN-γ and IL-15 that activate downstream auto-reactive CD8+ cells via JAK-STAT pathways. The autoreactive CD8+ cells also release perifollicular IFN-γ, inducing MHC-I expression and leading to the collapse of the IP. Previously sequestered autoantigens become exposed to CD8+ T cells via erroneous presentation though these MHC-I molecules. A secondary autoimmune phenomenon is triggered by the release of substance P from the hair follicles, which in conjunction with IFN-γ inhibits further hair growth.

be protective [53]. AA patients and murine models have been found to have fewer T regulatory cells and impaired CD4+CD25+ T regulatory cell function [54,55]. Xing et al. [56] demonstrated increased expression of certain polymorphisms with NKG2D receptor ligands in the hair follicle and infiltrating CD8+NKG2D+ T cells in affected skin. They went on to demonstrate in a mouse model for AA that CD8+NKG2D+ cells are necessary for adoptive transfer of AA to a normal recipient. Costimulatory factors such as stress are thought to contribute to destruction of the IP via substance P and mast cell degranulation [3,57,58].

Genomic studies

There are over 100 single nucleotide polymorphisms (SNPs) associated with AA, most of which are found in genes that code for aspects of inflammation (see **Table 4.2**). Genome-wide association studies (GWAS) support the theories described in above by demonstrating common variants amongst AA patients in loci associated with regulatory T cells and natural killer cells expressing NKG2D [2].

Table 4.2: Selection of genes implicated in alopecia areata, all of varying significance, alongside their description, function and other disease associations [2,59] (adapted from Betz et al. 2015 and Petukhova et al. 2010)			
Function/description	**Gene**	**Associated conditions**	**Source**
Genes associated with immunoregulation			
T cell proliferation/regulation	IL-21/IL-2 (also B- and NK-cell proliferation)	T1DM, RA, CeD, PS	Petukhova et al. 2010
	CTLA4 CT60	RA	Megiorni et al. 2013 [60]
	IL-2RA	T1DM, MS, GD, V	Petukhova et al. 2010
Natural killer cell NKG2D activating ligand	ULPB6, ULBP3		Petukhova et al. 2010
	MICA	T1DM, RA, CeD, UC, PS, SLE	Petukhova et al. 2010
Regulatory T cell transcription/differentiation/function	FOXP3 and ICOSLG	MM	Conteduca et al. 2012 [61]
	Eos (IKZF4)	T1DM, SLE	Petukhova et al. 2010
	GARP (LRRC32)	Autoimmune and inflammatory diseases	Betz et al. 2015
JAK signalling	SH2B3(LNK)		Betz et al. 2015
Antigen presentation	HLA-DRA	T1DM, RA, CeD, MS, GV	Petukhova et al. 2010
	HLA-DQA1	T1DM, RA, CeD, MS, SLE, PS, CD, UC, GD	Petukhova et al. 2010
	HLA-DQA2	T1DM, RA	Petukhova et al. 2010
	HLA-DQB2	RA	Petukhova et al. 2010
Cytokine	IL13	PA, RA, A	Jagielska et al. 2012 [62]
Co-stimulatory family	CTLA4	T1DM, RA, CeD, MS, SLE, GD	Petukhova et al. 2010
	BTNL2	T1DM, RA, UC, CD, SLE, MS, V	Petukhova et al. 2010
	ICOS		Petukhova et al. 2010
Genes associated with end organ function			
Premature hair greying	STX17		Petukhova et al. 2010
Antioxidant enzyme	PRDX5	MS	Petukhova et al. 2010
Other/unknown			
Tyrosine phosphatase	PTPN22	T1DM, RA, SLE, HT GD, AD, MG, V, SS, JIA, PA	Burn et al. 2011 [63] Kemp et al. 2006 [64] Salinas-Santander et al. 2015 [65]
Epidermal growth factor receptor	ERBB3	T1DM, SLE	Petukhova et al. 2010
Acyl-coenzyme A oxidase family (ACOXL) Apoptosis and autophagy regulation [BCL2L11(BIM)]	ACOXL/BCL2L11(BIM)	IgAN, PSC, T1DM	Betz et al. 2015
Haematopoeitic differentiation	NOTCH4	T1DM, RA, MS	Petukhova et al. 2010
Unknown	C6orf10	T1DM, RA, PS, V	Petukhova et al. 2010
	KIAA0350	MS, T1DM	Jagielska et al. 2012

Transcript profiling by Xing et al. [56] has implicated members of the γ_c cytokine–receptor pathway and IFN-γ in AA. The involvement of these suggests a role for downstream signalling via JAK molecules. This is supported by gene expression data, which showed increased JAK1 and JAK3 expression in diseased human and mouse skin.

Abbreviations: ACOXL, Acyl-coenzyme A oxidase family; A, Asthma; CD, Crohn's disease; CeD, celiac disease; GD, Graves' disease; IgAN, immunoglobulin-A nephropathy; JIA, juvenile idiopathic arthritis; MG, myasthenia gravis; MM, multiple myeloma; MS, multiple sclerosis; PS, psoriasis; PSC, primary sclerosing cholangitis; PA, psoriatic arthritis; RA, rheumatoid arthritis; SLE, system lupus erythematosus; SS, systemic sclerosis; T1DN, type I diabetes; UC, ulcerative colitis; HT, Hashimoto's thyroiditis; AD, Addison's disease; V, vitiligo.

EMERGING THERAPEUTIC OPTIONS

The JAK-STAT signalling pathway

Topical and systemic application of JAK-STAT pathway inhibitors has been shown to successfully reverse AA and induce hair growth in murine and human studies [56,66]. Inhibition of the JAK-STAT pathway is a particularly attractive treatment target for AA as these treatments have the potential to be administered topically or orally.

There are three JAK-STAT pathway inhibitors of interest, namely tofacitinib, ruxolitinib and baricitinib. Ruxolitinib and tofacitinib have been shown to promote re-entry of the mouse hair follicle into anagen by activating the 'normal' anagen initiation signalling pathways [66].

Tofacitinib is an approved treatment for rheumatoid arthritis in the US and is undergoing phase III trials for treatment of psoriasis [67]. It is a JAK 1/3 inhibitor that has been shown to have an effect on both the innate and adaptive immune responses [68]. Case studies of treatment with oral Tofacitinib have reported outcomes with varying degrees of success [69–71]. Craiglow et al. [69] reported almost total hair regrowth after 8 months of treatment in a male patient with AA universalis taking oral tofacitinib for this and his co-existent psoriasis. In a subsequent phase II trial of 66 patients treated with 5 mg oral tofacitinib, 32% experienced an improvement of 50% or more [72]. The most commonly experienced adverse reactions were mild infections. Response to treatment at 3 months follow up indicates that its effects might be transient, and a further phase II trials of oral tofacitinib is under way [73]. Oral tofacitinib may have additional benefits as it has been shown to improve AA-related nail disease in one case report [74]. A recent clinical trial in Yale reported on the efficacy of topical tofacitinib as a potential treatment. Its study showed that the level of response to topical tofacitinib is less than seen with oral tofacitinib but is similar to that reported with topical steroids under occlusion. Further studies are necessary to better understand JAK inhibitor treatment of AA [75].

Ruxolitinib, a JAK 1/2 inhibitor, is already in use for the treatment of myelofibrosis [76]. Mackay-Wiggan et al. [77] performed a phase II pilot study on the response to oral ruxolitinib in patients with moderate to severe AA. Of the 12 patients, the majority showed significant hair regrowth and downregulation of inflammatory markers. Adverse effects include mild skin, respiratory and urinary tract infections, anaemia and mild gastrointestinal symptoms. An additional case study suggests that oral treatment with an alternative JAK 1/2 inhibitor, baricitinib, may also be beneficial in AA [78].

Table 4.3 Summary of studied new therapeutic options for alopecia areata [107] (adapted from Falto-Aizpurua et al. 2014)			
Compound	Application	Mechanism of action	Summary of evidence
Ruxolitinib	Oral	JAK-STAT pathway inhibitors	Pilot study (phase II)
Tofacitinib	Oral Topical	Ruxolitinib and Baricitinib = JAK 1/2 inhibitor Tofacitinib = JAK 1/3 inhibitor	One phase II trial, case reports
Baricitinib	Oral		One case report
Platelet rich plasma	Intravenous	Contains and releases through degranulation several growth factors and cytokines	Two RCT Smaller non-RCT
Interleukin-2	Subcutaneous	Induce T-cell proliferation. An impaired inhibitory function of circulating CD4+CD25+ regulatory T cells has been reported to play a key role in AA	Prospective open ended
Abatacept	Subcutaneous	Blocks co-stimulation of T cells and reduces levels of TNF-α and interferon gamma	Preclinical mice studies with human studies currently underway
Bimatoprost	Topical	Prostglandin analogue	Nonblinded RCT
Excimer laser	Topical	Decreased T cell depletion and decreased antigen presentation	Five nonrandomised trials
Bexarotene	Topical	Selectively activates retinoid X receptors	One phase I/II randomised single blind trial
Hydroxychloroquine	Oral	Immunomodulatory effects	Case series
Capsaicin	Topical	Unknown	One pilot study
Simvastatin/ezetimibe	Oral	Lymphocytic modulators	One prospective pilot study
Triamcinolone	Intramuscular	Immunosuppression	One retrospective study

Abbreviations: RCT, randomised controlled trial; TNF-α, tumour necrosis factor-alpha; AA, alopecia areata; JAK-STAT, Janus kinase/signal transducer and activator of transcription;

Platelet-rich plasma

Platelet-rich plasma (PRP) therapy consists of growth-factor-rich platelets in concentrated plasma. It is being increasingly used in medicine in the fields of orthopaedics, sports medicine, dentistry and dermatology and has received significant media attention because of its promise as a regenerative therapy [79]. In vitro and in vivo studies have shown that it can promote hair survival and growth [80,81]. It is usually obtained by drawing blood from the patient, centrifuging, separating the PRP fraction and suspending it in calcium gluconate and then re-administering the PRP to the patient using an aseptic technique, however can also be less preferentially be sourced from a donor. PRP is known to carry more than twenty growth factors that are thought to work synergistically to induce inflammation, cell proliferation, differentiation and regeneration [82].

Smaller non-randomised studies and case reports have shown mixed results and further larger studies are required to determine its efficacy [83,85]. The first RCT to assess the efficacy of PRP on hair growth in patients with chronic recurring AA was performed by Trink et al. and published in 2013 [86]. Forty-five patients were randomised to one of three groups: PRP, triamcinolone acetonide 2.5 mg/mL or placebo. Changes in alopecia severity using the SALT score were statistically significant in favour of the PRP treatment group and it was also found to decrease hair dystrophy. Ki-67 levels, a marker for cellular proliferation, were found to be highest in the PRP treated group.

A recent larger RCT performed in 90 patients evaluated the efficacy of PRP versus minoxidil 5% versus placebo [87]. Results showed significant hair growth in 81% of those with patchy alopecia in the minoxidil group, 70% in the PRP group and 30% in the placebo group. The authors state that the PRP group showed a significant decrease in short vellus hair, yellow dots and dystrophic hairs as well as having an earlier hair growth response.

Interleukin 2

Interleukin 2 (IL-2) is a pleiotropic cytokine that has been found to induce T-cell proliferation. An impaired inhibitory function of circulating CD4+CD25+ regulatory T cells plays a key role in AA. The US Food and Drug Administration (FDA) have approved recombinant IL-2 (aldesleukin) for the treatment of metastatic renal cell cancers.

In a prospective open-ended study performed in five patients with severe AA resistant to previous systemic treatments, four patients achieved partial regrowth [88] after subcutaneous IL-2 administration. The primary outcome was the evolution of the SALT score. No serious adverse events were experienced; however there were reports of asthenia, arthralgia, urticarial and local reactions at injection sites.

Abatacept

Abatacept (CTLA4-Ig) targets T-cell activation and is currently used in the treatment of rheumatoid arthritis and juvenile idiopathic arthritis [89]. Preclinical mice studies showed promise in the treatment of AA and a phase II human study has been undertaken but results are pending [90,91].

Bimatoprost

Synthetic prostamides like bimatoprost were initially designed to reduce intraocular pressure for the treatment of glaucoma but have also been found to induce hypertrichosis. Bimatoprost's exact mechanism of action in hair growth is unknown, however, it is thought to work by promoting and prolonging anagen [92,93]. Bimatoprost 0.03% solution has been approved by the FDA for eyelash hypotrichosis. With regards to scalp AA, a nonblinded randomised clinical study involving 30 patients were assigned to treatment with either mometasone furoate 0.1% cream once daily or bimatoprost 0.03% twice daily for 3 months [94]. Results showed that the bimatoprost group demonstrated better results regarding percentage of hair re-growth, side effects and rapidity of response in weeks measured by reduction in SALT score.

Excimer laser

Excimer laser is a form of ultraviolet laser that emits monochromatic UVB light at a wavelength of 308 nm. Some clinical studies have documented the efficacy of excimer laser and excimer light in AA. In one controlled study, 41.5% patches were shown to respond to excimer laser therapy administered over 12 weeks [95]. Another study on childhood AA found regrowth in 60% lesions after a treatment period of 12 weeks [96]. The treatment is generally well tolerated with erythema of the skin as the only adverse effect reported.

Topical bexarotene

Bexarotene is a retinoid which when used in the treatment of patients with follicular mucinosis or folliculotropic mycosis fungoides yielded significant hair regrowth. In a phase I/II randomised single blind trial bexarotene was applied to one side of the scalp of 42 patients with varying degrees of severity of AA (34 with patchy AA, 3 with alopecia totalis and 5 with alopecia universalis). 12% of participants exhibited at least 50% hair regrowth on the treated side of the scalp. However, an additional 14% of patients had regrowth on both sides of the scalp [97], therefore further research is needed.

Hydroxychloroquine

Hydroxychloroquine is an antimalarial that is thought to have immunomodulatory effects. An initial study published in 2013 demonstrated improvement in refractory alopecia totalis in two patients treated with 200 mg twice daily was noted [98]. Unfortunately, a larger case series published in 2016 involving eight patients with alopecia totalis and extensive AA failed to demonstrate any lasting regrowth [99].

Capsaicin

Capsaicin is an active component of chilli peppers and is thought to release substance P, a neuropeptide that is implicated in AA. Based on the results of a pilot study of two patients and a small randomised trial, topical capsaicin may be able to stimulate vellus hair growth, however a cosmetically significantly hair growth has not been demonstrated [100].

Simvastatin/ezetimibe

Simvastatin with ezetimibe is a drug combination used for the treatment of dyslipidaemia. They also have immunomodulatory effects [101], with Simvastatin thought to act by suppressing MHC II expression [102]. A prospective study showed that 14 of 19 participants experienced at least 20% hair regrowth after treatment with this combination and nine had at least 70% hair regrowth [103]. This was sustained in a second phase of the study for five of seven patients who continued treatment for an additional 24 weeks, although one patient experienced hair loss and one was lost to follow-up. Positive response in this study was determined by 20% hair regrowth after 6 months. Treatment benefit is also described in a case report [104], however, a prospective pilot study involving 17 patients with severe AA totalis/universalis or >70% scalp involvement was less promising. Of the 17 patients, 14 (82%) had no hair regrowth, 2 (12%) had transient diffuse hair regrowth followed by total hair loss and 1 (6%) had patchy hair regrowth that was not cosmetically acceptable. Side effects including mild headache or muscle cramps that did not interrupt treatment were reported in three patients [105].

Intramuscular triamcinolone

In a retrospective study performed on 27 South Korean patients with refractory AA (defined as an unsatisfactory response to both systemic treatment and DPCP immunotherapy) were treated with intramuscular triamcinolone for 3–6 months. This resulted in a 63% response rate and the authors reported that all patients showed inactive disease after treatment. They also report that all patients showed complete recovery of adrenocortical reserve within 3 months after the last injection. However, adverse effects such as dysmenorrhea and osteoporosis were noted in female patients [106].

CONCLUSION

Alopecia areata is a disease affecting an increasing number of people yet despite causing significant morbidity current treatment options are unsatisfactory. Commonly used regimes include treatments that have significant side effect profiles, high relapse rates and disappointing results. Animal models and genetic studies are guiding the search for novel targets, and at present there are more than 10 studied treatment options that are summarised below. At present none of these are being used in regular clinical practice, but the landscape of AA management is changing.

Key points for clinical practice

- Intralesional steroid is treatment of choice for discrete patches of alopecia covering a limited area of scalp.

- Systemic therapy with corticosteroid can be effective for more widespread alopecia but should be administered with adjuvant systemic immunosuppressive agents such as ciclosporin, methotrexate or azathioprine to prevent relapse.

- Oral JAK kinase inhibitors have been shown to be effective in the treatment of alopecia areata in published cases. further trials will indicate if this will become a safe and effective treatment for wider use.

REFERENCES

1. Villasante Fricke AC, Miteva M. Epidemiology and burden of alopecia areata: a systematic review. Clin Cosmet Investig Dermatol 2015; 8:97–403.
2. Betz RC, Petukhova L, Ripke S, et al. Genome-wide meta-analysis in alopecia areata resolves HLA associations and reveals two new susceptibility loci. Nat Commun 2015; 6:5966.
3. Gilhar A, Schrum AG, Etzioni A, Waldmann H, Paus R. Alopecia areata: Animal models illuminate autoimmune pathogenesis and novel immunotherapeutic strategies. Autoimmun Rev 2016; 15:726–735.
4. Ikeda T. A new classification of alopecia areata. Dermatologica 1965; 131:421–445.
5. Delamere FM, Sladden MM, Dobbins HM, Leonardi-Bee J. Interventions for alopecia areata. Cochrane Database Syst Rev 2008:CD004413.
6. Olsen EA. Investigative guidelines for alopecia areata. Dermatol Ther 2011; 24: 311–319.
7. Messenger AG, McKillop J, Farrant P, McDonagh AJ, Sladden M. British Association of Dermatologists' guidelines for the management of alopecia areata 2012. Br J Dermatol 2012; 166:916.
8. Olsen EA, Hordinsky MK, Price VH, et al. National Alopecia Areata Foundation. Alopecia areata investigational assessment guidelines – Part II. J Am Acad Dermatol 2004; 51:440–447.
9. Charuwichitratana S, Wattanakrai P, Tanrattanakorn S. Randomized double-blind placebo-controlled trial in the treatment of alopecia areata with 0.25% desoximetasone cream. Arch Dermatol 2000; 136:1276.
10. Tosti A, Piraccini BM, Pazzaglia M, Vincenzi C. Clobetasol propionate 0.05% under occlusion in the treatment of alopecia totalis/universalis. J Am Acad Dermatol 2003; 49:96–98.
11. Walsh P, Aeling JL, Huff L, Weston WL. Hypothalamus-pituitary-adrenal axis suppression by superpotent topical steroids. J Am Acad Dermatol 1993; 29:501.
12. Keipert JA, Kelly R. Temporary Cushing's syndrome from percutaneous absorption of betamethasone 17-valerate. Med J Aust 1971; 1:542
13. Khaitan BK, Mittal R, Verma KK. Extensive alopecia areata treated with betamethasone oral mini-pulse therapy: an open uncontrolled study. Indian J Dermatol Venereol Leprol 2004; 70:350–353.
14. Yeo IK, Ko EJ, No YA, et al. Comparison of High-Dose Corticosteroid Pulse Therapy and Combination Therapy Using Oral Cyclosporine with Low-Dose Corticosteroid in Severe Alopecia Areata. Ann Dermatol 2015; 27:676–681.
15. Wiseman MC, Shapiro J, MacDonald N, Lui H. Predictive model for immunotherapy of alopecia areata with diphencyprone. Arch Dermatol 2001; 137:1063–1068.

16. Aghaei S. Topical immunotherapy of severe alopecia areata with diphenylcyclopropenone (DPCP): experience in an Iranian population. BMC Dermatol 2005; 5:6.
17. Rokhsar CK, Shupack JL, Vafai JJ, Washenik K. Efficacy of topical sensitizers in the treatment of alopecia areata. J Am Acad Dermatol 1998; 39:751–761.
18. Mitchell AJ, Douglass MC. Topical photochemotherapy for alopecia areata. J Am Acad Dermatol 1985; 12:644–649.
19. Taylor CR, Hawk JL. PUVA treatment of alopecia areata partialis, totalis and universalis: audit of 10 years' experience at St John's Institute of Dermatology. Br J Dermatol 1995; 133:914.
20. Fenton DA, Wilkinson JD. Topical minoxidil in the treatment of alopecia areata. Br Med J 1983; 287: 1015–17.
21. Price VH. Double-blind, placebo-controlled evaluation of topical minoxidil in extensive alopecia areata. J Am Acad Dermatol 1987; 16:730.
22. Vestey JP, Savin JA. A trial of 1% minoxidil used topically for severe alopecia areata. Acta Derm Venereol 1986; 66:179–80.
23. Price VH, Willey A, Chen BK. Topical tacrolimus in alopecia areata. J Am Acad Dermatol 2005; 52:138–139.
24. Nelson DA, Spielvogel RL. Anthralin therapy for alopecia areata. Int J Dermatol. 1985; 24:606–607.
25. Fiedler-Weiss VC, Buys CM. Evaluation of anthralin in the treatment of alopecia areata. Arch Dermatol 1987; 123:1491–1493.
26. Hay IC, Jamieson M, Ormerod AD. Randomized trial of aromatherapy. Successful treatment for alopecia areata. Arch Dermatol 1998; 134:1349–1352.
27. Willemsen R, Haentjens P, Roseeuw D, Vanderlinden J. Hypnosis in refractory alopecia areata significantly improves depression, anxiety, and life quality but not hair regrowth. J Am Acad Dermatol 2010; 62:517–518.
28. Strober BE, Siu K, Alexis AF, et al. Etanercept does not effectively treat moderate to severe alopecia areata: an open-label study. J Am Acad Dermatol 2005; 52:1082–1084.
29. Strober BE, Menon K, McMichael A, et al. Alefacept for severe alopecia areata: a randomized, double-blind, placebo-controlled study. Arch Dermatol 2009; 145:1262–1266.
30. Ferran M, Calvet J, Almirall M, Pujol RM, Maymo J. Alopecia areata as another immune-mediated disease developed in patients treated with tumour necrosis factor-alpha blocker agents: report of five cases and review of the literature. J Eur Acad Dermatol Venereol 2011; 25:479–484.
31. Joly P. The use of methotrexate alone or in combination with low doses of oral corticosteroids in the treatment of alopecia totalis or universalis. J Am Acad Dermatol 2006; 55:632–636.
32. Anuset D, Perceau G, Bernard P, Reguiai Z. Efficacy and Safety of Methotrexate Combined with Low- to Moderate-Dose Corticosteroids for Severe Alopecia Areata. Dermatology 2016; 232:242–248.
33. Hammerschmidt M, Mulinari Brenner F. Efficacy and safety of methotrexate in alopecia areata. An Bras Dermatol 2014; 89:729–734.
34. Droitcourt C, Milpied B, Ezzedine K, et al. Interest of high-dose pulse corticosteroid therapy combined with methotrexate for severe alopecia areata: a retrospective case series. Dermatology 2012; 224:369–373.
35. University Hospital, Rouen. The Efficiency Of The Methotrexate At Patients Affected By Grave Pelade (MP3). Clinicaltrials.gov 2016.
36. Gupta AK, Ellis CN, Cooper KD, Nickoloff BJ, Ho VC, Chan LS, Hamilton TA, Tellner DC, Griffiths CE, Voorhees JJ. Oral cyclosporine for the treatment of alopecia areata. A clinical and immunohistochemical analysis. J Am Acad Dermatol 1990; 22:242–250.
37. Lee D, Oh DJ, Kim JW, et al. Treatment of Severe Alopecia Areata: Combination Therapy Using Systemic Cyclosporine A with Low Dose Corticosteroids. Ann Dermatol 2008; 20:172–178.
38. Shaheedi-Dadras M, Karami A, Mollaei F, Moravvej H, Malekzad F. The effect of methylprednisolone pulse-therapy plus oral cyclosporine in the treatment of alopecia totalis and universalis. Arch Iran Med 2008; 11:90–93.
39. Kim BJ, Min SU, Park KY, et al. Combination therapy of cyclosporine and methylprednisolone on severe alopecia areata. J Dermatolog Treat 2008; 19:216–220.
40. Açıkgöz G, Calışkan E, Tunca M, Yeniay Y, Akar A. The effect of oral cyclosporine in the treatment of severe alopecia areata. Cutan Ocul Toxicol 2014; 33:247–252.
41. Cerottini JP, Panizzon RG, de Viragh PA. Multifocal alopecia areata during systemic cyclosporine A therapy. Dermatology 1999; 198:415–417.
42. Dyall-Smith D. Alopecia areata in a renal transplant recipient on cyclosporin. Australas J Dermatol 1996; 37:226–227.

43. Phillips MA, Graves JE, Nunley JR. Alopecia areata presenting in 2 kidney-pancreas transplant recipients taking cyclosporine. J Am Acad Dermatol 2005; 53:S252–255.
44. Park KY, Jang WS, Son IP, et al. Combination therapy with cyclosporine and psoralen plus ultraviolet a in the patients with severe alopecia areata: a retrospective study with a self-controlled design. Ann Dermatol 2013; 25:12–16.
45. Kim BJ, Min SU, Park KY, et al. Combination therapy of cyclosporine and methylprednisolone on severe alopecia areata. J Dermatolog Treat 2008; 19:216–220.
46. Gilhar A, Pillar T, Etzioni A. Topical cyclosporin A in alopecia areata. Acta Derm Venereol 1989; 69:252–253.
47. Rongioletti F, Guarrera M, Tosti M, Guerra L, Pigatto P. Topical cyclosporin A fails to improve alopecia areata – a double blind study. J Dermatol Treat 1992; 3:13–14.
48. Nelson B, Ratner D, Weiner N, et al. Efficacy of topical cyclosporin a in the treatment of alopecia areata. J Dermatol Treat 1994; 5:77–79.
49. Guerra N, Pestal K, Juarez T, et al. A selective role of NKG2D in inflammatory and autoimmune diseases. Clin Immunol 2013; 149: 432–439.
50. Billingham RE, Silvers WK. A biologist's reflections on dermatology. J Invest Dermatol 1971; 57:227–240.
51. Paus R, Nickoloff BJ, Ito T. A 'hairy' privilege. Trends Immunol 2005; 26:32–40.
52. Wang, EH, Yu M, Breitkopf T, et al. Identification of Autoantigen Epitopes in Alopecia Areata. J Invest Dermatol 2016; 136:1617–1626.
53. McElwee KJ, Freyschmidt-Paul P, Hoffmann R, Kissling S, Hummel S, Vitacolonna M, Zoller M. Transfer of CD8(+) cells induces localized hair loss whereas CD4(+)/CD25(-) cells promote systemic alopecia areata and CD4(+)/CD25(+) cells blockade disease onset in the C3H/HeJ mouse model. J Invest Dermatol 2005; 124:947–957.
54. Castela E, Le Duff F, Butori C, et al. Effects of low-dose recombinant interleukin 2 to promote T-regulatory cells in alopecia areata. JAMA Dermatol 2014; 150:748–751.
55. Shin BS, Furuhashi T, Nakamura M, Torii K, Morita A. Impaired inhibitory function of circulating CD4+CD25+ regulatory T cells in alopecia areata. J Dermatol Sci 2013; 70:141–143.
56. Xing L, Dai Z, Jabbari A, et al. Alopecia areata is driven by cytotoxic T lymphocytes and is reversed by JAK Inhibition. Nat Med 2014; 20:1043–1049.
57. Siebenhaar F, Sharov AA, Peters EM, et al. Substance P as an immunomodulatory neuropeptide in a mouse model for autoimmune hair loss (alopecia areata). J Invest Dermatol 2007; 127:1489–1497.
58. Peters EM, Liotiri S, Bodó E, et al. Probing the effects of stress mediators on the human hair follicle: substance P holds central position. Am J Pathol 2007; 171:1872–1886.
59. Petukhova L, Duvic M, Hordinsky M, et al. Genome-wide association study in alopecia areata implicates both innate and adaptive immunity. Nature 2010; 466:113–117.
60. Megiorni F, Mora B, Maxia C, et al. Cytotoxic T-lymphocyte antigen 4 (CTLA4) +49AG and CT60 gene polymorphisms in Alopecia Areata: a case-control association study in the Italian population. Arch Dermatol Res 2013; 305:665–670.
61. Conteduca G, Rossi A, Megiorni F, et al. Single nucleotide polymorphisms in the promoter regions of Foxp3 and ICOSLG genes are associated with alopecia areata. Clin Exp Med 2014; 14:91–97.
62. Jagielska, D, Redler S, Brockschmidt FF. Follow-up study of the first genome-wide association scan in alopecia areata: IL13 and KIAA0350 as susceptibility loci supported with genome-wide significance. J Invest Dermatol 2012; 132:2192–2197.
63. Burn GL, Svensson L, Sanchez-Blanco C, Saini M, Cope AP. Why is PTPN22 a good candidate susceptibility gene for autoimmune disease? FEBS Lett 2011; 585:3689–3698.
64. Kemp EH, McDonagh AJ, Wengraf DA, et al. The non-synonymous C1858T substitution in the PTPN22 gene is associated with susceptibility to the severe forms of alopecia areata. Hum Immunol 2006; 67:535–539.
65. Salinas-Santander M, Sánchez-Domínguez C, Cantú-Salinas C, et al. Association between PTPN22 C1858T polymorphism and alopecia areata risk. Exp Ther Med 2015; 10:1953–1958.
66. Harel S, Higgins CA, Cerise JE, et al. Christiano AM. Pharmacologic inhibition of JAK-STAT signaling promotes hair growth. *Science Advances* 2015; 1:e1500973.
67. Gupta AK, Cernea M, Lynde CW. Tofacitinib in the Treatment of Rheumatoid Arthritis and Chronic Plaque Psoriasis. Skin Therapy Lett 2017; 22:1–7.
68. Ghoreschi K, Jesson MI, Li X, et al. Modulation of Innate and Adaptive Immune Responses by Tofacitinib (CP-690,550). J Immunol 2011; 186:4234–4243.
69. Craiglow BG, King BA. Killing two birds with one stone: oral tofacitinib reverses alopecia universalis in a patient with plaque psoriasis. J Invest Dermatol 2014; 134:2988–2990.

70. Gupta, AK, Carviel, JL, Abramovits, W. Efficacy of tofacitinib in treatment of alopecia universalis in two patients. J Eur Acad Dermatol Venereol 2016; 30:1373–1378.
71. Anzengruber F, Maul JT, Kamarachev J, et al. Transient efficacy of tofacitinib in alopecia areata universalis. Case Rep Dermatol 2016; 8:102–106.
72. Kennedy Crispin M, Ko JM, Craiglow BG, et al. Safety and efficacy of the JAK inhibitor tofacitinib citrate in patients with alopecia areata. JCI Insight 2016; 1:e89776.
73. Mackay-Wiggan J. Study to evaluate the efficacy of tofacitinib in moderate to severe alopecia areata, totalis and universalis. ClinicalTrials.gov 2017:NCT02299297.
74. Ferreira SB, Scheinberg M, Steiner D, et al. Remarkable Improvement of Nail Changes in Alopecia Areata Universalis with 10 Months of Treatment with Tofacitinib: A Case Report. Case Rep Dermatol 2016; 8:262–266.
75. Liu LY, Craiglow BG, King BA. Tofacitinib 2% ointment, a topical Janus Kinase inhibitor, for the treatment of alopecia areata: a pilot study of 10 patients. J Am Acad Dermatol. 2018; 78(2): 403-404.
76. Mesa RA. NCCN Debuts New Guidelines for Myeloproliferative Neoplasms. J Natl Compr Canc Netw 2017; 15:720–722.
77. Mackay-Wiggan J, Jabbari A, Nguyen N, et al. Oral ruxolitinib induces hair regrowth in patients with moderate-to-severe alopecia areata. JCI Insight 2016; 1:e89790.
78. Jabbari A, Dai Z, Xing L, et al. Reversal of Alopecia Areata Following Treatment With the JAK1/2 Inhibitor Baricitinib. EBioMedicine 2015; 2:351–355.
79. Keene DJ, Alsousou J, Willett K. How effective are platelet rich plasma injections in treating musculoskeletal soft tissue injuries? BMJ 2016; 352:517.
80. Li ZJ, Choi HI, Choi DK, et al. Autologous platelet-rich plasma: a potential therapeutic tool for promoting hair growth. Dermatol Surg 2012; 38:1040–1046.
81. Rogers N. Commentary on Autologous platelet-rich plasma: A potential therapeutic tool for promoting hair growth. Dermatol Surg 2012; 38:1047–1048.
82. Marie-Angeliki G, Alexandros-Efstratios K, Dimitris R, Konstantinos K. Platelet-rich plasma as a potential treatment for noncicatricial alopecias. Int J Trichology 2015; 7:54–63.
83. Khan S, Kamal T, Ellahi A, Ahmad TJ. Role of autologous platelet rich plasma (PRP) in limited alopecia areata in local population. J Pakistan Associat Dermatol 2016; 26:107–111.
84. Singh S. Role of platelet-rich plasma in chronic alopecia areata: Our centre experience. Indian J Plast Surg 2015; 48:57–59.
85. Mubki T. Platelet-rich plasma combined with intralesional triamcinolone acetide for the treatment of alopecia areata: a case report. J Dermatol Dermatol Surg 2016; 20:87–90.
86. Trink A, Sorbellini E, Bezzola P, et al. A randomized, double-blind, placebo- and active-controlled, half-head study to evaluate the effects of platelet-rich plasma on alopecia areata. Br J Dermatol 2013; 169:690–694.
87. El Taieb MA, Ibrahim H, Nada EA, Seif Al-Din M. Platelets rich plasma versus minoxidil 5% in treatment of alopecia areata: A trichosopic evaluation. Dermatologic Ther 2016; 30.
88. Castela E, Le Duff F, Butori C, et al. Effects of low-dose recombinant interleukin 2 to promote T-regulatory cells in alopecia areata. JAMA Dermatol 2014; 150:748–751.
89. Barut K, Adrovic A, Şahin S, Kasapçopur Ö. Juvenile Idiopathic Arthritis. Balkan Med J 2017; 34:90–101.
90. Sundberg JP, McElwee KJ, Carroll J, King LE. Hypothesis Testing: CTLA4 Co-Stimulatory Pathways Critical in the Pathogenesis of Human and Mouse Alopecia Areata. J Invest Dermatol 2011; 131:2323–2324.
91. Mackay-Wiggan J. An Open-Label Single-Arm Clinical Trial to Evaluate The Efficacy of Abatacept in Moderate to Severe Patch Type Alopecia Areata. ClinicalTrials.gov. 2016:NCT02018042.
92. Tauchi M, Fuchs TA, Kellenberger AJ, Woodward DF, Paus R, Lütjen-Drecoll E. Characterization of an in vivo model for the study of eyelash biology and trichomegaly: mouse eyelash morphology, development, growth cycle, and anagen prolongation by bimatoprost. Br J Dermatol 2010; 162:1186–1197.
93. Cohen JL. Enhancing the growth of natural eyelashes: the mechanism of bimatoprost-induced eyelash growth. Dermatol Surg 2010; 36:1361–1371.
94. Zaher H, Gawdat HI, Hegazy RA, Hassan M. Bimatoprost versus Mometasone Furoate in the Treatment of Scalp Alopecia Areata: A pilot study. Dermatology 2015; 230:308–313.
95. Al-Mutairi N. 308-nm excimer laser for the treatment of alopecia areata. Dermatol Surg 2007; 33:1483–1487.
96. Al-Mutairi N. 308-nm excimer laser for the treatment of alopecia areata in children. Pediatr Dermatol 2009; 26:547–550.

97. Talpur R, Vu J, Bassett R, Stevens V, Duvic M. Phase I/II randomized bilateral half-head comparison of topical bexarotene 1% gel for alopecia areata. J Am Acad Dermatol 2009; 61:592–598.

98. Stephan F, Habre M, Tomb R. Successful treatment of alopecia totalis with hydroxychloroquine: Report of 2 cases. J Am Acad Dermatol 2013; 68:1048–1049.

99. Nissen C, Wulf H. Hydroxychloroquine is ineffective in treatment of alopecia totalis and extensive alopecia areata: A case series of 8 patients. JAAD Case Rep 2016; 2:117–118.

100. Ehsani AH, Toosi S, Seirafi H, et al. Noormohamadpour P, Ghanadan A. Capsaicin vs. clobetasol for the treatment of localized alopecia areata. J Eur Acad Dermatol Venereol 2009; 23:1451–1453.

101. Tie, C, Gao, K, Zhang, N, et al. Ezetimibe Attenuates Atherosclerosis Associated with Lipid Reduction and Inflammation Inhibition. PLoS One 2015; 10:e0142430.

102. Kwak B, Mulhaupt F, Veillard N, Pelli G, Mach F. The HMG-CoA reductase inhibitor simvastatin inhibits IFN-gamma induced MHC class II expression in human vascular endothelial cells. Swiss Med Wkly 2001; 131:41–46.

103. Lattouf C, Jimenez J, Tosti A. Treatment of alopecia areata with simvastatin/ezetimibe. J Am Acad Dermatol 2015; 72:359–361.

104. Ali A, Martin JM. Hair growth in patients alopecia areata totalis after treatment with simvastatin and ezetimibe. J Drugs Dermatol 2010; 9:62–64.

105. Loi C, Starace M, Piraccini B. Alopecia areata and treatment with simvastatin/ezetimibe: Experience of 20 patients. J Am Acad Dermatol 2016; 74:99–100.

106. Seo J, Lee YI, Hwang S, Zheng Z, Kim DY. Intramuscular triamcinolone acetonide: An undervalued option for refractory alopecia areata. J Dermatol 2017; 44:173–179.

107. Falto-Aizpurua L, Choudhary S, Tosti A. Emerging treatments in alopecia. Expert Opin Emerg Drugs 2014; 19:545–556.

Chapter 5

What's new in contact allergy to cosmetics?

Eirini E Merika, Sarah H Wakelin

INTRODUCTION

Modern cosmetics are intended to be safe for users and strict regulations exist to ensure quality control with testing before release of new products onto the market. However, despite these measures, cosmetic allergy is frequently encountered in dermatology practice. The commonest allergens are fragrances, preservatives and hair dyes. Other allergens include antioxidants, emulsifiers, surfactants and humectants some of which may also be found in topical pharmaceutical products[1]. Natural ingredients, especially essential oils, are well recognised to cause allergy and can be found in products labelled as 'organic' or 'fragrance-free,' which can mislead consumers regarding their safety. Allergy to nail products is becoming commoner with the increasing popularity and availability of acrylic resins. Dermatologists play a key role in identifying new allergens and changes in the rate of allergy to existing allergens. The regulatory agencies need to respond promptly to this information in order to protect consumers from harm, but the legislative processes can be slow and cumbersome.

Allergic contact dermatitis (ACD) from cosmetics and toiletries usually affects the face and /or hands, but other affected areas include the axillae and anogenital area and in some cases the dermatitis may be generalised. Photoallergic contact dermatitis is relatively rare and involves the interaction of sunlight, particularly UVA, with the cosmetic ingredient, typically a sunscreen. The diagnosis of ACD is made by taking a careful history, thorough examination of the skin and performing diagnostic patch tests with additional photopatch tests for suspected photoallergy. The baseline series of allergens or 'standard series' should be supplemented with a cosmetics and toiletries series and testing with the patient's own skin care products, diluted if necessary. Repeat open application testing or usage testing can be helpful in cases of doubt. This involves application of the leave-on cosmetics or rinsed cosmetic to a localised area such as the elbow flexure twice a day for up to 3 weeks and observing the skin for a papular, eczematous reaction.

It is important to keep test series up to date to detect emerging allergens. This chapter provides an overview of recent trends in cosmetic contact allergy including the methylisothiazolinone (MI) 'epidemic,' terpene fragrance allergy, oxidative hair dyes and nail acrylates.

Eirini E Merika MBBS, BSc, MRCP (UK), MRCP (Derm) Consultant Dermatologist, Chelsea & Westminster Hospital NHS Foundation Trust, London, UK. Email: Eirini.Merika@doctors.org (for correspondence)

Sarah H Wakelin BSc, MBBS, FRCP Consultant Dermatologist & Honorary Senior Lecturer in Dermatology, Imperial College Healthcare NHS Trust, London, UK

PRESERVATIVES AND THE METHYLISOTHIAZOLINONE 'EPIDEMIC'

After fragrances, preservatives are the commonest group of cosmetic allergens. These include biocidal chemicals added to prevent the growth of micro-organisms. All biocides are potential sensitisers. Isothiazolinones, formaldehyde, formaldehyde-releasers, iodoproponylbutyl carbamate and parabens are the most commonly used agents among those permitted for use in cosmetics. Methyldibromoglutaronitrile was banned from use as a cosmetic preservative in Europe in 2007 after causing high rates of sensitisation in the 1990s. Unfortunately, history has repeated itself and in the last decade there has been an 'epidemic' of allergy to another biocide, MI with rates of allergy to this chemical far exceeding any other preservative reported so far. How did this happen?

Methylisothiazolinone was originally used in a 1:3 mixture with methylchlorisothiazolinone (MCI) as a biocide in cosmetics, toiletries, household goods and industrial products. The mix was marketed under various trade names including Kathon, Kathon CG, and Euxyl K100 and was recognised as a cause of cosmetic and occupational allergy with steady levels reported in the 1990s [2]. In 2005, changes to European legislation permitted use of MI alone at much higher concentrations of up to 100 parts per million (ppm), i.e. 0.01%, in leave-on and rinse off cosmetics. Just prior to this, there had been reports of occupational allergy to MI, mainly from paint exposure. The first reports ACD to MI, as a cosmetic and toiletry allergen in wet wipes was reported in 2010 [1]. Reports of florid cases of facial, anogenital, and generalised dermatitis from exposure to MI in cosmetics, toiletries and baby wet wipes followed, some making newspaper and television headlines. Indeed, over last 6 years there has been an unprecedented rise in the rates of MI allergy in patch test populations with rates of over 10% reported in the UK, mostly related to personal care products [4,5]. After repeated lobbying by dermatologists, European regulations were amended to prohibit the use of MI in leave-on cosmetics from the end of 2016 and reduce the concentration of MI permitted in rinse-off products to 15 ppm (0.0015%); a level considered to be safe for the induction of contact allergy [6].

Isothiazolinones are volatile and severe cases of airborne ACD have been reported among painters and consumers from exposure to water based paints. High airborne levels of MI, exceeding the ACD elicitation threshold, may occur for weeks after indoor painting. Unusual sources of exposure to MI include ironing water and adhesive labels (see Box 5.1). Photoaggravated contact dermatitis to MI/MCI mix has also been reported [7,8]. Because of its presence in diverse items, some of which are not yet ingredient labelled, patients who are allergic to MI remain at risk of inadvertent exposure despite attempted allergen avoidance.

Box 5.1 Common exposure sources for MI and MI/MCI

- *Personal care products:* Soap, bubble bath and shower gels, wet and dry baby wipes, shampoos (mostly zinc pyrithione-based anti-dandruff shampoos) and conditioners, hair products, skin creams and body lotions and sunscreens, mouth washes, mascaras, eyeshadows, make-up removers
- *Household products:* Detergents, fabric softeners, washing up liquid, ironing water, glues, polishes, water colours, household paints
- *Industrial products:* Car polish, wind screen products, glues and adhesives, cutting oils, cooling fluids, ECG electrode gels, pesticides, curing agents, printing inks

Methylisothiazolinone is included in the current European baseline series at a concentration of 2000 ppm, i.e. 0.2% in aqueous solution whereas MI/MCI mix is tested as a 0.01% aqueous solution. The higher test concentration of MI is needed to identify false negatives from testing with MI/MCI mix alone as the latter has been estimated to miss approximately 40% of cases of allergy to MI [9].

Sensitisation to MI has been reported to lead to cross reactivity to other isothiazolinones such as octylisothiazolinone, which is used as a preservative in household and industrial products and has recently been identified in leather clothing items [10]. High concentrations of isothiazolinones have been found in detergents which may therefore continue to pose a risk to consumers [11]. Continued monitoring of rates of allergy to MI in patch test populations will therefore play an important role in determining the effectiveness of the recent cosmetic regulations.

Fragrances

Fragrances are the commonest allergens in cosmetics and toiletries. As almost all skin care products and household products are fragranced, consumers are exposed to multiple sources in daily life. Emollients and topical medications such as barrier creams, nappy rash remedies, moisturisers, topical steroids and haemorrhoid preparations may also contain fragrance. Although fragrances are typically weak or moderate skin sensitisers, cumulative exposure is thought to give rise to fragrance allergy rates of approximately 2% in the general population [12]. ACD may follow direct skin application, close contact with another individual who wears fragranced products or airborne exposure.

There are several thousand fragrance chemicals which are natural, synthetic or derived from essential oils. Amendments in the European Directive on Cosmetic Products in 2003 and household products in 2005 has helped consumers identify some of the major allergens by specifying a list of 26 fragrances that have to be individually listed in the ingredients if the content exceeds 10 ppm in leave on and 100 ppm for rinse-off products (see **Box 5.2**). This list includes the 8 fragrance allergens of fragrance mix I (FM I) and the 6 of fragrance Mix II (FM II) which are used for screening in the European baseline series along with the natural plant extract Myroxylon pereirae (Balsam of Peru). Hydroxyisohexyl 3-cyclohexene carboxaldehyde (HICC), commonly referred to as 'lyral,' is also now included in the baseline series as a single allergen at a higher concentration than in FM II. These allergens/mixes clearly do not screen for all the 26 labelled fragrances however (see below), and a study of 281 patch test patients who were screened with all 26 individual fragrances reported that over 40% of those reacting to this extended fragrance series would have been missed by testing to the European baseline series alone. This included patients who reacted to FM I or FM II constituents but not the relevant mixes [13].

Despite these shortcomings, high rates of fragrance allergy have been detected in patch test populations. A large 29-year cross-sectional registry study in Denmark found that 7.8% (24,168 patients) were sensitised to FM I with most cases considered clinically relevant (78%). The rates of allergy increased with age in women and were higher in those with facial dermatitis [14]. Children may also be affected and similar rates of sensitisation have been noted in atopic and nonatopic individuals [15]. A large multi-centre retrospective analysis of 1142 paediatric patch test in the United States identified allergy to FMI in 11% and Balsam of Peru in 8.4% [16]. Fragrance allergy may cause occupational ACD with diverse sources of exposure sources including cutting oils and coolants. A large UK study reported that fragrance allergy accounted for 4.6% of 18943 cases of occupational ACD between

1996–2015. The majority of affected individuals were employed in healthcare, the beauty industry and food industry [17].

Box 5.2 Fragrances which are individually listed on EU cosmetics and toiletries

- *Fragrance mix I ingredients:* Cinnamic alcohol, cinnamic aldehyde, hydroxycitronellal, amylcinnamaldehyde, geraniol, euginol, isoeuginol, and oakmosse absolute
- *Fragrance mix II ingredients:* Lyral, citral, citronellol, farnesol, coumarin and hexyl cinnamic aldehyde
- *Others:* Alpha-isoethyl ionone, amylcinnamyl alcohol, anisyl alcohol, benzyl benzoate, cinnamate and salicylate, lilial (betylphenyl methylpropional), tree moss (evernia furfuracea) and methyl 2-octynoate

---

Essential oils

Essential oils are natural extracts from plants and flowers and are frequently used as fragrances in perfumery, medicine and aromatherapy. Over 80 essential oils have been reported to have caused contact allergy usually when applied in their pure forms or at high concentration [18].

Of all essential oils, tea tree oil allergy has been reported most commonly with a patch test prevalence ranging from 0.1–35% [19]. The other essential oils most frequently reported as sensitisers are ylang-ylang oil, lemongrass oil, jasmine absolute, sandalwood oil and clove oil [20]. The risk of sensitisation is highest in aromatherapists and masseuses due to repeated skin exposure. Unsuspected sources of fragrance include medicaments, e.g. a recent report highlighted the presence of balsam of pine in fluocinolone oil used to treat scalp dermatitis with improvement on avoiding all balsam containing products [21].

Limonene and linalool

Terpenes are a large class of volatile organic compounds, and major constituents of plant and flower essential oils, particularly those from confiners. They often have a strong aroma and are used as fragrances and flavourings. Limonene and linalool are among the commonest naturally-occurring terpenes and have been identified in more than 200 essential oils (See **Box 5.3**). Limonene has a citrus aroma whereas linalool smells of lavender. They are included in the EU list of 26 specified fragrances (see above) and can be found prestige perfumes, personal care products (e.g. aftershave lotions, deodorants, shampoo and conditioners, mouthwashes), household products (e.g. detergent, air fresheners, cleaning products and botanical insecticides) and industrial products. It is important to remember that they are not individually listed as ingredients when they exist in the form of an essential oil.

Limonene and linalool are not considered to be allergenic in their pure forms, but they undergo auto-oxidation on exposure to air forming various oxides and peroxides which are potent sensitisers. Sensitised individuals may therefore not react to new or recently-opened products that contain unoxidised fragrances. Positive patch test rates to oxidised R-limonene of 2–3% have been reported among consecutive patch tested patients [22]. Testing with 3% oxidised R-limonene in petrolatum with stable limonene hydroperoxides (0.33%) is considered to be the most useful patch test reagent, with an average detection rate of 5.2% (range 2.3–12.1%) in a series of 2900 tested[23]. Likewise allergy to oxidised R-linalool has been detected in 5% of consecutive patch test patients [24]. Oxidised linalool 6% with stable linalool hydroperoxides (1%) is considered to be the optimal patch test reagent, with a detection rate ranging from 3–13% [24,25]. Given these relatively high rates of allergy inclusion of these allergens is recommended in the extended UK baseline series [26].

Concomitant allergy to both oxidised limonene and linalool is not frequent and when present, is thought to represent sensitisations from difference fragrance materials in consumer products [27].

Box 5.3: Essential oils that contain limonene and linalool

- *Linalool containing oils:* Lavender, cinnamon, ylang-ylang, bergamot, jasmine, geranium, rosewood, coriander, orange and lemon zest, basil, laurel
- *Limonene containing oils:* Citrus, lavender, geranium bergamot, rosewood, tea tree and plant oils

---

Oxidative hair dyes

The majority of permanent and semi-permanent chemical (oxidative) hair dyes contain para-phenylene diamine (PPD) or related amines. These have been used for over 100 years and are clearly recognised to be potent sensitisers and a hazard to health, to such a degree that they have been banned in several European countries at varying times. It is estimated that over 40,000,000 salon applications of hair dye are carried out in the UK and a similar, if not higher, number of home hair colorants are sold each year [28]. It has been estimated that the rate of allergy to PPD is approximately 1% in health populations in Germany [29]. Several reports from the last decade have highlighted increasing rates of PPD sensitisation among Europe patch test populations [30]. In London alone there has been a doubling in the frequency of ACD to PPD in the last 6 years to 7% [30]. A 12-year review of PPD contact allergy in Europe identified 99,926 positive reactions (4%), 50–75% of which were likely to be considered to be clinically relevant [30].

The precise allergen is thought to be an oxidation product of PPD rather than PPD itself. There may be a spectrum of antigenic determinants including 4-nitroaniline and 4,4'-azodianiline which have both been shown to be potent sensitisers [32]. Once fully oxidised, PPD is no longer a sensitiser which explains why PPD allergic patients can wear dyed clothing items.

ACD to PPD in hair dye typically presents with a relapsing chronic dermatitis of the scalp, hair margin or ear tips. Hair dye is also used to darken eyebrows, lashes and beards. Sensitised individuals typically develop localised ACD within half a day to a few days of application of the dye. Current EU legislation permits PPD at a concentration of up to 6% concentration in consumer hair dye. The addition of PPD to henna for skin and nail painting ('henna tattoos'/ 'black henna') represents an illegal use and alarmingly high concentrations of up to 30% PPD have been reported [22,23]. These are associated with a very high risk of sensitisation. One study reported an odds ratio of 9.33 for development of PPD allergy following exposure to black henna [12]. Moreover, sensitisation by skin painting is also associated with severe allergic dermatitis on subsequent use of hair dye with florid swelling of the face and scalp mimicking angioedema, i.e.'pseudoangioedema'. There have also been rare reports of genuine immediate-type allergy and anaphylaxis following use of PPD dyes.

Sensitisation is lifelong and may lead to cross reactions with other dyes, drugs and sunscreens. Occupational allergy to PPD is a considerable problem among hairdressers causing chronic hand dermatitis, sickness leave and ultimately loss of employment. Confusion can arise from misleading labelling of hair colourants branded as 'organic' or 'natural' as these can contain PPD or derivatives which may not be listed on the label [34].

There is a high rate of cross-reaction between PPD and other chemically related dyes, especially p-toluenediamine, aminophenols and azo dyes. P-toluenediamine has been recommended as suitable alternative to PPD-positive patients on the grounds that 50% of PPD allergic individuals were able to tolerate the dye [35]. However, they remain at risk of subsequent sensitisation with ongoing use. Aware of the clear need to develop safer hair colourants, a group of manufacturers have recently published date on use of 2-methoxymethyl-PPD (ME-PPD) which is proposed as a less sensitising alternative. Early studies indicate tolerance of ME-PPD colourants in approximately 65–70% of PPD/PTD allergic patients [36]. However, these have involved relatively small numbers of volunteers and careful dermatological evaluation will be required to assess the real-life tolerability of these dyes.

Nail cosmetics

Nail cosmetics include varnishes and polishes (enamels), enamel removers, cuticle removers and artificial nails. ACD and irritant dermatitis may occur following contact with these agents and can present with fingertip dermatitis ('pulpitis'), paronychia, nail dystrophy and onycholysis. Ectopic ACD at other body sites, especially eyelids and neck and the vulva may occur. Nail enamels contain of film formers, resins, plasticisers, solvents, colourants and pearlisers. The most common reagent responsible for allergic reactions to enamels is tosylamide formaldehyde resin, which has been recognised as an allergen since the 1940s. Enamel and cuticle removers usually cause irritant contact dermatitis because of their high solvent concentration. 'Hypoallergenic' nail varnish based on polyester resin or cellulose acetate butyrate can also sensitise and tend to be less durable than tosylamide enamel. Newer nail varnish allergens include acrylate copolymers, phthalic anhydride/trimellitic anhydride [37], but the rates of allergy to these are unknown as they are not yet routinely available as patch test allergens.

Nail acrylates

Historically ACD to acrylates was related to occupational exposure in dentists, printers, painters and fibreglass workers. Following the increased popularity of artificial nails, extensions and nail enhancements which utilise acrylate or methacrylate chemicals, ACD is now being reported most frequently in nail technicians and consumers. Rates are likely to increase further given the increasing availability of home kits. Acrylate allergy has been reported to affect over 10% of selected UK patch test populations and at least 2% of all consecutively patch tested patients [38]. Nail acrylates were nominated as 'contact allergen of the year' for 2012 by the American Contact Dermatitis Society. The most common presentation is finger pulp and periungual dermatitis, but paraesthesiae, sensory loss, decreased dexterity, onycholysis and nail shedding have also been reported. Facial dermatitis, rhinoconjunctivitis and allergic asthma may also occur.

Acrylates and methacrylates exist as monomers in powder, liquids, pastes or gels. During polymerisation they become pliable before hardening or 'curing'. When fully polymerised they are usually nonirritant or allergenic. Nail technicians are at highest risk of sensitisation due to frequent exposure to unpolymerised monomers. Some acrylates polymerise spontaneously in air, others require exposure to ultraviolet (UV) radiation [39]. The most common acrylates used in the acrylic nail industry are liquid methacrylate acid esters, such as ethyl methacrylate, hydroxyethyl acrylate, 2-hydroxyethyl methacrylate (2-HEMA), n-(2-hydroxypropyl)methacrylate (2-HPMA), ethylene glycol dimethacrylate (EGDMA) and powdered polymethyl ethacrylate.

Cyanoacrylates or 'superglues' such as ethyl-cyanoacrylate (ECA) are also used as adhesives as they polymerise quickly and strongly on exposure to moisture. They are used to stick artificial nails to the underlying nail plate ('nail tips') and are also used as an adhesive for false eyelashes ('lash extensions'). Contact allergy relatively rare because of their rapid polymerisation. They are also used medically as skin glues and in household instant glues. Acrylates such as ECA can cause permanent damage the nail plate with dystrophy or nail loss.

The term 'sculptured nails' or 'gel nails' refer to a custom-made blend of chemicals including UV-cured acrylates which are applied to the prepared nails, surrounded by a template that protects the surrounding skin, to form artificial extensions. Gels are brushed onto the nails in three steps: base coat, polish colour and top coat. Each coat has to be cured by UV light. 'Shellac' refers to an increasingly popular form of long-lasting nail polish which is a blend of acrylic gel and nail polish. Home UV sources are now commercially available, but improper use can lead to incomplete exposure of the resin and risk of consumer exposure to sensitising monomers. Nail technicians and beauticians may also lack training and awareness of the risk of allergy to themselves and customers: A large retrospective analysis of acrylate patch test results among 114,440 patients tests identified 47.1% sensitisation rate in 87 nail technicians [40]. In another study a 'mini-acrylate' series identified 16/241 (6.6%) positive patch test reactions all of which were thought to be relevant, the majority being occupational [41]. Simultaneous allergy to 2-HEMA, EGMA and 2-HPA is also common as are cross-reactions and even cross-sensitisation amongst acrylates. A short acrylate series comprising methyl methacrylate, 2-HEMA, ethyl acrylate, ethylene dimethacrylate, triethylene glycol diacrylate, and ethyl cyanoacrylate will identify most nail acrylate allergic individuals. Testing with HEMA alone has been reported to detect most cases. Patch test allergens must be prepared freshly before testing as acrylates are volatile and pre-prepared patches can give false negative results. Nail chemicals containing (meth)acrylate monomers should never be applied to skin undiluted because of the risk of sensitisation.

Occupational protection should involve use of adequate gloves such as tri-laminated polyethylene or nitrile gloves. Natural rubber latex and vinyl are not suitable as they are rapidly penetrated by methyl methacrylate.

Sunscreens

Chemicals which function as UV filters are widely used in sunscreens and facial cosmetics for their sun protective effects. They are also added to toiletries to prevent photodegradation. Modern sunscreens typically contain a combination of UV filters in order to achieve broad spectrum cover and these can cause both ACD and more rarely, photo-ACD. In addition, they usually contain other common allergens such as fragrances and preservatives. The investigation of suspected sunscreen allergy therefore requires patch testing and photopatch testing. Photopatch test series need to be updated with the emergence of new photocontact allergens. The patient's own sunscreens should also be tested.

Benzophenones are primarily UVB absorbers, though benzophenone-3 (oxybenzone) and benzophenone-4 (sulisobenzone) also absorb UVAII, hence their widespread use. Benzophenone-3 is the leading allergen and photocontact allergen and is included in the British baseline series. Dibenzoyl methanes and tinosorb M are also the most commonly implicated UV filters. Octocrylene is a relatively new UVB and UVAII absorber that was introduced 15 years ago and is now widely used. It has been reported as a relatively frequent contact allergen in children due to its use in sunscreens and has also emerged as a photoallergen in adults, especially those with a history of photoallergy to the nonsteroidal anti-inflammatory drug ketoprofen, which cross reacts with benzophenone-3. The mechanism whereby photosensitisation to ketoprofen leads to photocontact allergy to octocrylene is unknown at present [42].

Para-aminobenzoic acid (PABA) was one of the first UVB sunscreens, but is rarely used nowadays as in addition to ACD and photo-ACD, it has been associated with other adverse reactions including irritancy and staining of clothing.

CONCLUSION

Cosmetics remain a common cause of ACD despite safety regulations. The culprit ingredients range from long established allergens such as fragrance and oxidative hair dyes to newer preservatives and nail acrylates. These pose a risk to consumers and beauty professionals. It is essential that clinicians remain informed of emerging allergens and that patch test series are updated accordingly. The diagnosis of cosmetic ACD involves taking a thorough, focused history and testing with supplemental allergens and the patient's own cosmetics, diluted when necessary. Correct and timely identification of allergens is also important to limit morbidity. It is only with continuous patient and public education and cosmetic industry scrutiny that cosmetic contact allergy will be kept at reasonable levels, if not diminish.

Key points for clinical practice

- The commonest allergens are fragrances, preservatives and hair dyes but allergy to acrylates is becoming increasingly common.

- MI has caused an 'epidemic' of ACD in consumers since 2005 following its inclusion in a wide range of cosmetics and toiletries. Other sources of exposure include household goods and industrial products, especially water based paints.

- Fragrances are the commonest allergens in skin care products. They include natural fragrances, essential oils and synthetic fragrances. Fragrance mix I and II does not detect all fragrance allergy; limonene and linalool are recommended for inclusion in the baseline patch test series. 'Natural' products may contain hidden fragrance allergens. Children are also at risk of developing fragrance allergy.

- PPD and its derivatives are strong sensitisers; black henna tattoos contain PPD and are associated with a high risk of lifelong sensitisation. New PPD derivatives are under investigation but their safety in consumer populations remains unproven.

- Acrylate allergy is a common cause of occupational and consumer ACD and may cause remote site reactions. Allergy is shifting from an occupational allergy to consumer allergy. Causative allergens may not be present in the usual patch test series. Test all ingredients and patients own products.

REFERENCES

1. Goossens A. Contact-allergic reactions to cosmetics. J Allergy (Cairo) 2011; 2011:467071.
2. Jacobs MC, White IR, Rycroft RJ, Taub N. Patch testing with preservatives at St John's from 1982 to 1993. Contact Dermatitis 1995; 33:247–254.
3. Garcia-Gavin J, Vansina S, Kerre S, Naert A, Goossens A. Methylisothiazolinone, an emerging allergen in cosmetics? Contact Dermatitis 2010; 63:96–101.
4. Venables ZC, Bourke JF, Buckley DA, et al. Has the epidemic of allergic contact dermatitis due to Methylisothiazolinone reached its peak? Br J Dermatol 2016; 177:276–278.
5. DeKoven JG, Warshaw EM, Belsito DV, et al. North American Contact Dermatitis Group Patch Test Results: 2013-2014. Dermatitis 2017; 28:33–46.
6. Methylisothiazolinone, quo vadis? Contact Dermatitis 2016; 75:263–264.
7. Pirmez R, Fernandes AL, Melo MG. Photoaggravated contact dermatitis to Kathon CG (methylchloroisothiazolinone/methylisothiazolinone): a novel pattern of involvement in a growing epidemic? Br J Dermatol 2015; 173:1343–1344.
8. Trokoudes D, Banerjee P, Fityan A, et al. Photoinduced and photoaggravated allergic contact dermatitis due to methylisothiazolinone. ESCD: Contact Dermatitis; 2017; 76:303–304.
9. Castanedo-Tardana MP, Zug KA. Methylisothiazolinone. Dermatitis 2013; 24:2–6.
10. Aerts O, Goossens A, Bervoets A, Lambert J. Almost Missed It! Photo-contact Allergy to Octocrylene in a Ketoprofen-sensitized Subject. Dermatitis 2016; 27:33–34.
11. Garcia-Hidalgo E, Sottas V, von Goetz N, et al. Occurrence and concentrations of isothiazolinones in detergents and cosmetics in Switzerland. Contact Dermatitis 2017; 76:96–106.
12. Diepgen TL, Naldi L, Bruze M, et al. Prevalence of Contact Allergy to p-Phenylenediamine in the European General Population. J Invest Dermatol 2016; 136:409–415.
13. Mann J, McFadden JP, White JM, White IR, Banerjee P. Baseline series fragrance markers fail to predict contact allergy. Contact Dermatitis 2014; 70:276–281.
14. Bennike NH, Zachariae C, Duus Johansen J. Trends in contact allergy to fragrance mix I in consecutive Danish eczema patients over three decades; a cross-sectional study from 1986 to 2015. Br J Dermatol 2017; 176:1035–1041.
15. Lubbes S, Rustemeyer T, Sillevis Smitt JH, Schuttelaar MA, Middelkamp-Hup MA. Contact sensitization in Dutch children and adolescents with and without atopic dermatitis – a retrospective analysis. Contact Dermatitis 2017; 76:151–159.
16. Goldenberg A, Mousdicas N, Silverberg N, et al. Pediatric Contact Dermatitis Registry Inaugural Case Data. Dermatitis 2016; 27:293–302.
17. Montgomery RL, Agius R, Wilkinson SM, Carder M. UK trends of occupatioal skin disease. ESCD: Contact Dermatitis 2016.
18. de Groot AC, Schmidt E. Essential Oils, Part IV: Contact Allergy. Dermatitis 2016; 27:170–175.
19. de Groot AC, Schmidt E. Tea tree oil: contact allergy and chemical composition. Contact Dermatitis 2016; 75:129–143.
20. Uter W, Schmidt E, Geier J, et al. Contact allergy to essential oils: current patch test results (2000-2008) from the Information Network of Departments of Dermatology (IVDK). Contact Dermatitis 2010; 63:277–283.
21. Admani S, Goldenberg A, Jacob SE. Contact Alopecia: Improvement of Alopecia with Discontinuation of Fluocinolone Oil in Individuals Allergic to Balsam Fragrance. Pediatr Dermatol 2017; 34:e57–e60.
22. Matura M, Goossens A, Bordalo O, et al. Oxidized citrus oil (R-limonene): a frequent skin sensitizer in Europe. J Am Acad Dermatol 2002; 47:709–714.
23. Brared Christensson J, Andersen KE, Bruze M, et al. An international multicentre study on the allergenic activity of air-oxidized R-limonene. Contact Dermatitis 2013; 68:214–223.
24. Brared Christensson J, Andersen KE, Bruze M, et al. Air-oxidized linalool: a frequent cause of fragrance contact allergy. Contact Dermatitis 2012; 67:247–259.
25. Brared Christensson J, Andersen KE, Bruze M, et al. Positive patch test reactions to oxidized limonene: exposure and relevance. Contact Dermatitis 2014; 71:264–272.
26. Audrain H, Kenward C, Lovell CR, et al. Allergy to oxidized limonene and linalool is frequent in the UK. Br J Dermatol 2014; 171:292–297.
27. Brared Christensson J, Karlberg AT, Andersen KE, et al. Oxidized limonene and oxidized linalool – concomitant contact allergy to common fragrance terpenes. Contact Dermatitis 2016; 74:273–280.
28. Krasteva M, Bons B, Tozer S, et al. Contact allergy to hair colouring products. The cosmetovigilance experience of 4 companies (2003–2006). Eur J Dermatol 2010; 20:85–95.

29. Schnuch A, Lessmann H, Frosch PJ, Uter W. para-Phenylenediamine: the profile of an important allergen. Results of the IVDK. Br J Dermatol 2008; 159:379–386.
30. Patel S, Basketter DA, Jefferies D, et al. Patch test frequency to p-phenylenediamine: follow up over the last 6 years. Contact Dermatitis 2007; 56:35–37.
31. Schuttelaar ML, Vogel TA, Rui F, et al. ESSCA results with the baseline series, 2002-2012: p-phenylenediamine. Contact Dermatitis 2016; 75:165–172.
32. Young E, Zimerson E, Bruze M, Svedman C. Two sensitizing oxidation products of p-phenylenediamine patch tested in patients allergic to p-phenylenediamine. Contact Dermatitis 2016; 74:76–82.
33. Al-Suwaidi A, Ahmed H. Determination of para-phenylenediamine (PPD) in henna in the United Arab Emirates. Int J Environ Res Public Health 2010; 7:1681–1693.
34. Thoren S, Yazar K. Contact allergens in 'natural' hair dyes. Contact Dermatitis 2016; 74:302–304.
35. Scheman A, Cha C, Bhinder M. Alternative hair-dye products for persons allergic to para-phenylenediamine. Dermatitis 2011; 22:189–192.
36. Blomeke B, Pot LM, Coenraads PJ, et al. Cross-elicitation responses to 2-methoxymethyl-p-phenylenediamine under hair dye use conditions in p-phenylenediamine-allergic individuals. Br J Dermatol 2015; 172:976–980.
37. Gach JE, Stone NM, Finch TM. A series of four cases of allergic contact dermatitis to phthalic anhydride/trimellitic anhydride/glycols copolymer in nail varnish. Contact Dermatitis 2005; 53:63–64.
38. Rajan S, Orton DI, Chowdhury MM, et al. Contact allergy to (meth)acrylates: a U.K. multicentre study. Contact Dermatitis Special Issue: 13th Congress of the European Society of Contact Dermatitis (ESCD), 14–17 September 2016, Manchester, UK 2016; 75:2078–2085.
39. Ramos L, Cabral R, Goncalo M. Allergic contact dermatitis caused by acrylates and methacrylates – a 7-year study. Contact Dermatitis 2014; 71:102–107.
40. Uter W, Geier J. Contact allergy to acrylates and methacrylates in consumers and nail artists – data of the Information Network of Departments of Dermatology, 2004-2013. Contact Dermatitis 2015; 72:224–228.
41. Muttardi K, White IR, Banerjee P. The burden of allergic contact dermatitis caused by acrylates. Contact Dermatitis 2016; 75:180–184.
42. de Groot AC, Roberts DW. Contact and photocontact allergy to octocrylene: a review. Contact Dermatitis 2014; 70:193–204.

Chapter 6

Advances in atopic eczema

Teresa Tsakok, Richard Woolf, Carsten Flohr

INTRODUCTION

Atopic eczema (synonym 'atopic dermatitis', 'eczema') is one of the commonest chronic inflammatory skin disorders, affecting up to 20% of children and 5% of adults in industrialised countries [1]. Approximately 40% of childhood cases persist into adulthood, affecting work productivity and social functioning, and the associated impact on quality of life is comparable to having epilepsy or type 1 diabetes [2]. Thus atopic eczema represents a considerable burden to both the individual and society. It has been estimated to cost the UK more than £806 million a year (adjusted for inflation) [3], and up to US$5 billion annually in the USA [4].

The pathophysiology of atopic eczema is complex, encompassing both genetic risk factors and multiple environmental triggers. It has long been established that dysregulation of innate and adaptive immunity plays a key role, and the traditional paradigm of atopic eczema espouses a Th2-skewed immune system with exaggerated IgE responses to environmental allergens. However, recent findings from epidemiological and molecular research have focused interest on skin barrier dysfunction as a common precursor and pathological feature. Genome wide association studies (GWAS) have identified over 30 susceptibility loci, with the strongest known genetic risk factor being a mutation in the gene that encodes the epidermal protein filaggrin [5]. Current understanding of the aetiology of atopic eczema highlights disruption of the epidermal barrier leading to increased permeability of the epidermis, pathological inflammation in the skin, and percutaneous sensitisation to allergens. Thus, most novel treatment strategies seek to specifically target aspects of the skin barrier or cutaneous inflammation. In addition, several recent studies have shown promise in preventing atopic eczema, such as the use of early emollients in high-risk infants. This may have broader implications in terms of halting the progression of the so-called 'atopic march', thereby preventing the development of associated atopic comorbidities such as food allergy, hay fever, and asthma.

Teresa Tsakok, NIHR Academic Clinical Fellow and Specialty Trainee in Dermatology, St John's Institute of Dermatology, King's College London, London, UK

Richard Woolf, NIHR Academic Clinical Lecturer and Specialty Trainee in Dermatology, St John's Institute of Dermatology, King's College London, London, UK

Carsten Flohr*, Reader and Head, Unit for Population-Based Dermatology Research, St John's Institute of Dermatology, King's College London, London, UK, Email: carsten.flohr@kcl.ac.uk (for correspondence).

In this chapter, we review recent advances in our understanding of the pathogenesis of atopic eczema, and show how these are driving the development of targeted strategies in treatment and prevention.

CLINICAL FEATURES AND DIAGNOSIS

Atopic eczema presents clinically as ill-defined erythematous, scaly and pruritic patches of skin inflammation. These morphological features reflect underlying pathological changes, including the infiltration of lymphocytes and granulocytes, the development of epidermal oedema (spongiosis), and often secondary bacterial infection.

Despite our increased understanding of the molecular pathology of atopic eczema, it remains a clinical diagnosis. Several diagnostic criteria define key features of the condition, including those of Hanifin and Rajika [6], and the extensively validated UK Working Party diagnostic criteria [7]. Patients must have a history of itchy skin, plus at least three of the following: a history of flexural involvement (e.g. folds of the elbows or backs of the knees); visible flexural dermatitis; a personal history of other atopic disease (asthma or hay fever), or in a first degree relative if aged <4 years; history of generally dry skin (xerosis) in the last year; and onset of symptoms before the age of 2 years [7].

In most children and adults, atopic eczema typically affects the flexures (**Figure 6.1**); however, eczema can affect any body site. For example, atopic eczema in infants and patients with racially pigmented skin commonly involves nonflexural sites such as the face and limbs, whereas atopic eczema in adults may extend from flexural sites to involve the hands and neck – particularly if exacerbated by environmental irritants.

In addition, atopic eczema is associated with an increased propensity to form IgE antibodies to common allergens. Subsequent exposure to these allergens in sensitised

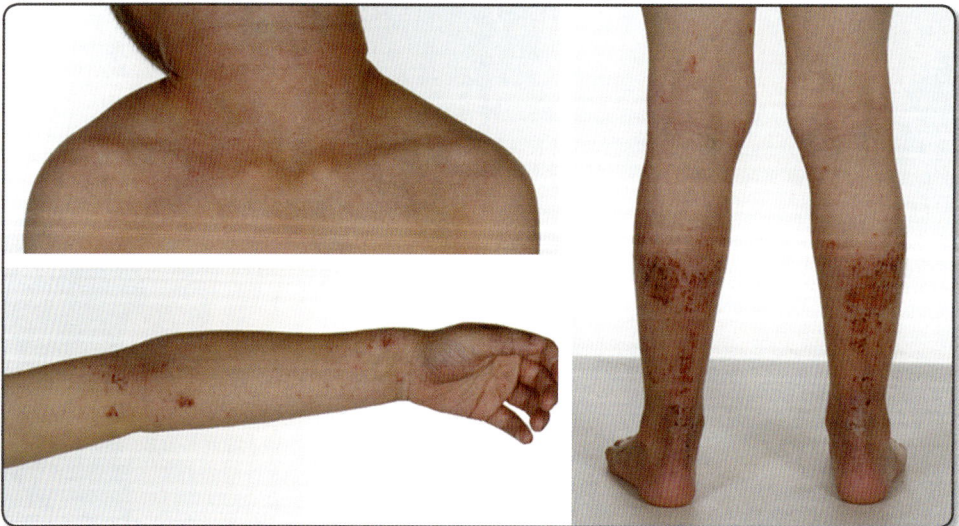

Figure 6.1 Atopic eczema in a child, affecting not only flexural (neck and antecubital fossa) but also nonflexural areas (lower legs) with widespread excoriation from scratching. The yellow crusting suggests skin infection.

individuals can drive eczema flares and disease chronicity. Patients commonly report immediate hypersensitivity reactions and/or have elevated serum specific IgE levels, and this may form part of the diagnostic criteria.

Atopic eczema is also associated with a susceptibility to cutaneous infections, notably by bacteria such as *Staphylococcus aureus*, as well as certain viruses, including herpes simplex. Such secondary infections can complicate the clinical presentation and management of this condition.

SKIN BARRIER DYSFUNCTION

One of the most important functions of the skin, and in particular the epidermis, is to provide an effective barrier that protects against both dehydration and environmental insults. The structural and biochemical components of the skin barrier are complex, but a major constituent is the stratum corneum, which forms the outermost layer of the epidermis. Here keratinocytes have undergone apoptosis to become flattened 'squames' filled with keratin. Keratin filaments are tightly cross-linked by filaggrin molecules, and filaggrin degradation products are a source of natural moisturising factor in the so-called cornified envelope. The acidification of skin by filaggrin metabolites helps to maintain skin barrier integrity and a low skin pH, and conversely it appears that an increased skin pH stimulates protease activity and thereby contributes to skin barrier dysfunction [8].

In 2006, Palmer et al. published the seminal finding that loss-of-function mutations in the *FLG* gene were strongly associated with atopic eczema [9]. Filaggrin deficiency impacts on numerous pathways relevant for skin barrier function, such as disturbed keratinocyte differentiation, impaired corneocyte integrity and cohesion, impaired tight-junction formation, decreased water retention, stratum corneum acidification, altered lipid formation, and enhanced cutaneous infectivity [10]. This lent support to the 'outside-in' hypothesis that functional disruption of the epidermal barrier is the primary pathogenic process in atopic eczema, facilitating recognition of various environmental allergens, irritants and microbes, and thereby initiating a cascade of inflammatory events. *FLG* null mutations have since been found in many ethnic groups and represent the strongest known genetic risk factor for atopic eczema, increasing the risk by a factor of approximately four compared to the normal population. Furthermore, *FLG* null mutations predispose to earlier disease onset, prolonged duration and increased severity [11].

Nevertheless, reported frequencies of *FLG* mutations range only from 18–48% in eczema patients, and the population-attributable risk is only around 15% [12], implying that other cofactors also play an important role in the development of atopic eczema. For instance, cutaneous inflammation (predominantly Th2 cell mediated) [13] can cause a reduction in filaggrin expression in the skin – even in patients not carrying a *FLG* mutation. Apart from *FLG* mutations *per se*, the intragenic copy number of the *FLG* gene (typically 10–12 repeats) can independently affect atopic eczema risk, with an increased copy number being protective, approximately equating to a 12% reduction in risk for each *FLG* repeat [14]. Furthermore, the *FLG* gene is only one of a cluster of genes located on chromosome 1q21 that are involved in epidermal differentiation – the so-called epidermal differentiation complex (EDC). Alongside *FLG*, at least 45 genes are located in this EDC. Notably, accounting for *FLG* variation in a study investigating linkage to atopic eczema in a UK population did not eliminate the linkage peak in the 1q21 region, suggesting that additional EDC genes may contribute to atopic eczema pathogenesis [15]. One such gene encodes the protein hornerin, which is important for keratinocyte differentiation with similar functions to filaggrin. Hornerin is present in the epidermal cornified envelope, and levels of hornerin and other filaggrin-like proteins, such as filaggrin 2, are decreased in the skin of atopic eczema patients [16].

Deep to the cornified envelope, tight junctions in the granular layer form an additional component of the physical skin barrier. Tight junctions facilitate the paracellular passage of soluble mediators, and play a key role in regulating transepidermal water loss (TEWL). They are composed of transmembrane proteins, including the claudin family. Expression of claudin-1 is reduced in the skin of atopic eczema patients, and SNPs in the *CLDN1* gene have been associated with atopic eczema in two North American cohorts [17]. A reduction in claudin-1 may enhance viral penetration and thus increase susceptibility to eczema herpeticum [18].

Eczematous inflammation has also been associated with variation in the *SPINK5* gene encoding *LETKI1*, a protease inhibitor effective in the epidermis. In fact, loss of function mutations in *SPINK5* are critical in Netherton syndrome, a rare and severe autosomal recessive form of ichthyosis with secondary dermatitis. Further research into rare congenital disorders with an eczema-like phenotype, including Wiskott–Aldrich syndrome and hyper-IgE syndrome, may shed additional light on the pathogenesis of atopic eczema.

Recently, emerging evidence suggests that the defects in structural epidermal proteins described above may collectively contribute to systemic sensitisation via the skin. This in turn may lead to distal allergic inflammation in other tissues (e.g. the respiratory tract or gut), as well as flares in established atopic eczema, thus contributing to more severe and chronic disease. Palmer et al. were the first to make the observation that *FLG* mutation carriers have an increased risk of developing asthma, but only in the context of current or previous atopic eczema [9]. This has now been consistently replicated, and since then *FLG* mutations have also been found to be associated with aeroallergen sensitisation and hay fever, primarily in the context of early-life atopic eczema.

Since filaggrin is not expressed in respiratory epithelia, the most likely explanation is that transcutaneous sensitisation to aeroallergens occurs via an impaired epidermal barrier. A similar mechanism may apply to food sensitization [19]; for instance, infants with peanut allergy by the age of 5 years are more likely to have had severe atopic eczema in the first 6 months of life, and to have been treated with peanut oil for dry skin [20]. Another study comparing 71 challenge-proven peanut allergy patients with 1,000 nonsensitised controls found an almost four-fold increase in peanut allergy risk in children with at least one *FLG* mutation compared to wild-type children, even after adjustment for atopic eczema. The risk of peanut allergy almost doubled in children with atopic eczema in early life [21]. More recently, Brough et al. showed that high levels of peanut in household dust were associated with an increased risk of sensitisation and likely peanut allergy in children with atopic eczema. Importantly, this risk was augmented in children with more severe disease [22]. Finally, Flohr et al. showed independent links between skin barrier impairment (raised TEWL), atopic eczema phenotype, and food sensitisation as early as 3 months of age. Atopic eczema increased the risk of food sensitisation more than six-fold overall. There was also a stepwise increase in food sensitisation risk with more severe atopic eczema, even after adjustment for *FLG* mutation inheritance and TEWL [23].

Environment

Taken together, the evidence discussed above implies that atopic eczema is initiated by a defective skin barrier. Once the skin barrier is disrupted and inflamed, transcutaneous antigen exposure and allergic priming is facilitated by antigen-presenting cells in the epidermis (i.e. dendritic cells). Therefore, any environmental factor that has a detrimental effect on skin barrier integrity should consequently enhance atopic eczema risk. Mechanical damage, such as repetitive scratching, the use of detergents and the release of exogenous proteases (for instance from dust mite allergen) are all thought to contribute to loss of skin barrier integrity.

Controversy still surrounds the optimal bathing frequency to recommend to parents of children with atopic eczema. A recent review of the available evidence found that studies in favour of frequent bathing outnumber those in favour of infrequent bathing [24]. On a related note, a large UK birth cohort study has reported that high levels of hygiene at 15 months of age were independently associated with atopic eczema reported between 30–42 months, and there was also an increased risk for children with more severe atopic eczema during this period [25].

Climactic factors are also thought to be relevant. Recently, a merged analysis of the USA 2007 National Survey of Children's Health and the 2006–2007 National Climate Data Center and Weather Service found that atopic eczema prevalence was higher in areas with lower relative humidity, lower ultraviolet (UV) index, lower mean temperatures, higher precipitation and more indoor heating [26].

Finally, there is also increasing evidence to suggest that domestic water hardness is a modifiable risk factor for the development of atopic eczema. A recently published study amongst 1303 3-month-old infants from the general population in England and Wales gathered data on domestic water calcium carbonate and chlorine concentrations from local water suppliers. At enrolment, infants were examined for atopic eczema, screened for FLG mutation status, and TEWL was measured on unaffected skin. The authors reported that living in a hard water area was associated with an up to 87% increased risk of atopic eczema at 3 months of age, independent of domestic water chlorine content. The risk tended to be higher in children with mutations in the FLG skin barrier gene [27].

IMMUNOLOGY

In addition to skin barrier impairment, atopic eczema is defined by pathological inflammation within the skin (**Figure 6.2**). GWAS analyses [5] have identified multiple susceptibility loci that are associated with components of the innate and adaptive immune system, immune regulation and tissue responses. These findings are supported by mechanistic studies.

Impairment in epidermal barrier function may directly predispose to and trigger the cutaneous inflammation seen in atopic eczema. For instance, mice with a loss-of-function mutation in the FLG gene ('flaky tail' mice) develop a spontaneous atopic eczema-like dermatitis. Other work has shown that filaggrin deficiency is associated with increased epidermal permeability, enhanced percutaneous microbial and allergen penetration, and reduced inflammatory thresholds to irritants and haptens [28–30]. Damage to the epithelium – such as by repetitive scratching – leads to activation of innate immune mechanisms, including the release of proinflammatory cytokines and chemokines by keratinocytes (e.g. IL-1 family cytokines, thymic stromal lymphopoietin [TSLP], IL-25 and IL-31) [31,32], antigen presentation by nonprofessional antigen presenting cells (e.g. keratinocytes) [33], and antigen presentation by skin-resident Langerhans' cells and dermal dendritic cells via classical MHC or unconventional MHC-like pathways [30, 34] (**Figure 6.3**).

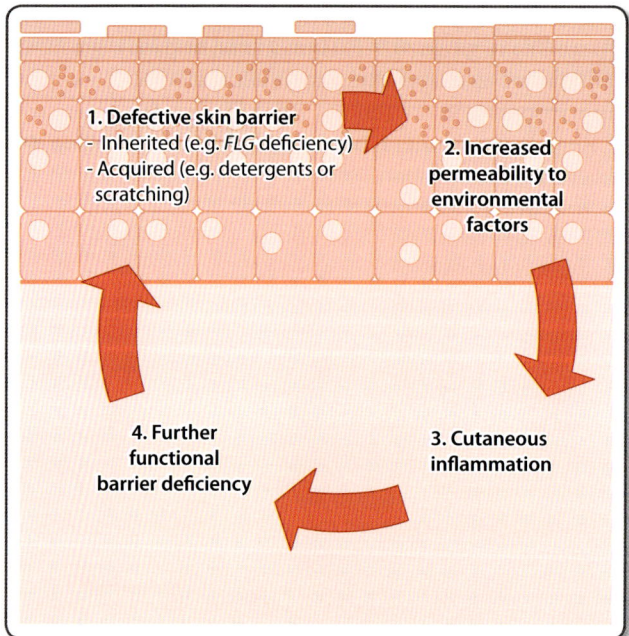

Figure 6.2 Atopic eczema cycle. Due to both inherited and acquired factors, a defective skin barrier predisposes to the development of cutaneous inflammation, which in turn causes further functional impairment in skin barrier function.

These events in turn initiate a proinflammatory cascade, characterised by the sequential and progressive infiltration of different inflammatory cell subsets. Atopic eczema is largely thought to be driven by CD4+ T helper 2 (Th2) cells, with cytokine release by damaged keratinocytes playing a key role in the context of antigen presentation and Th2 cell recruitment. Th2 lymphocytes are defined by their production of the cytokines interleukin (IL)-4, IL-5 and IL-13. Even 'nonlesional' skin in patients with atopic eczema shows signs of subclinical inflammation, with increased numbers of Th2 cells [35]. As active dermatitis develops, the skin becomes acutely infiltrated with more Th2 cells and additional CD4+ subsets, including Th22 and Th17 cells that secrete IL-22 and IL-17 respectively [36]. In addition to CD4+ T cells, other lymphocyte subsets are found in increased numbers within the infiltrate, and these include type 2 cytokine-producing CD8+ T cells and innate lymphoid cells (ILCs) [37,38]. The role of innate lymphocyte populations such as ILCs remains uncertain; however, they may have a key role in the early sensing of tissue damage and initiation of such inflammatory cascades, prior to the development of antigen-driven adaptive immune responses. Th2-like inflammation leads to the recruitment of additional immune cell subsets including eosinophils and mast cells, which further contribute to pathological inflammation through the release of mediators such as histamine.

In the chronic stages of atopic eczema, a more mixed inflammatory response can be observed, with recruitment of Th1 lymphocytes to the skin (defined by their production of interferon-γ (IFNγ)], leading to a mixed Th1, Th2 and Th22 infiltrate [35]. These activated lymphocytes adopt a tissue-resident memory T cell phenotype, meaning that they have limited capacity to recirculate out of the skin and are primed in the tissue, ready to mount rapid recall responses when re-exposed to antigenic triggers. Such disease-associated lymphocyte subsets in the skin may be cross-reactive to autoantigens or antigens commonly encountered at the epidermis (e.g. house dust mite and *Malasezzia furfur*) [39],

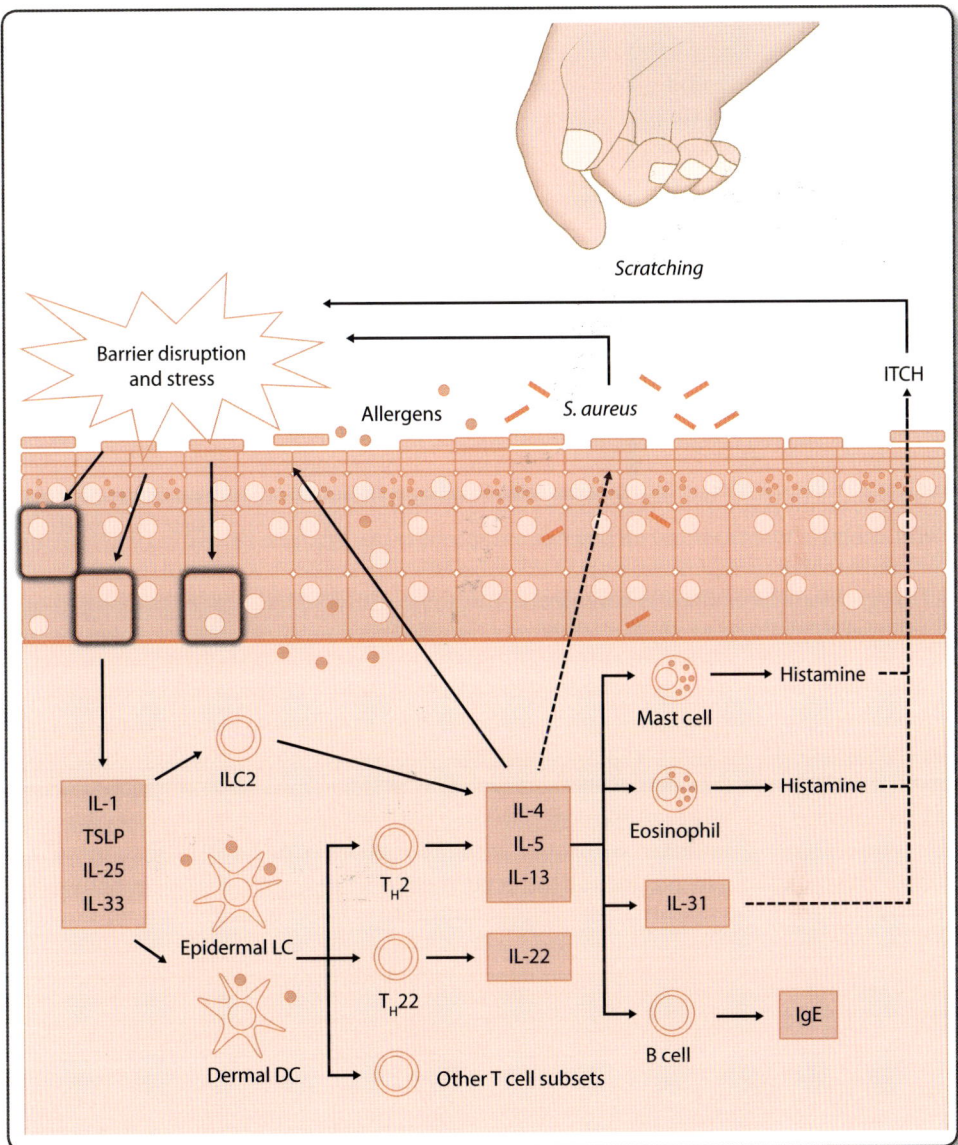

Figure 6.3 Immunopathogenesis of atopic eczema. Epidermal barrier dysfunction and stress from environmental factors is associated with increased epidermal permeability and enhanced microbial and allergen contact with the cutaneous immune system. Damaged epithelial cells activate innate immune mechanisms, such as the release of the proinflammatory cytokines IL-1, TSLP, IL-25 and IL-33, and additional chemokines. This leads to activation of innate lymphocyte subsets and antigen presenting cells, with subsequent T cell activation – atopic eczema is largely driven by CD4+ T helper 2 (Th2) cells, but other T cell subsets are found, including CD4+ Th22 cells. The type 2 cytokines IL-4, IL-5 and IL-13 drive further pathological changes, including eosinophil and mast cell recruitment and activation, B cell IgE production, and IL-31 secretion. There is also crosstalk between inflammatory cytokines, secreted molecules and cutaneous nerves to mediate pruritus, with resultant scratching causing further mechanical disruption of the skin barrier. The inflammatory environment also leads to further impairment in epidermal barrier function and favours S. aureus colonisation, leading to bacterial dysbiosis and positive reinforcement of the atopic eczema disease cycle.
Abbreviations: IL, interleukin; TSLP, thymic stromal lymphopoietin; Ig, immunoglobulin; TH, T helper cell, DC, dendritic cell; LC, Langerhans' cell; ILC, innate lymphoid cells.

and their persistence represents a major challenge in the treatment of chronic atopic eczema.

The pathogenesis of atopic eczema is further complicated by the interaction between skin inflammation and skin barrier function. It has become increasingly clear that inflammatory responses within the skin can in fact lead to widespread secondary changes that further contribute to the atopic eczema phenotype. Such effects include the suppression of epidermal differentiation genes, including filaggrin, loricrin, and involucrin by Th2, Th22 and Th1 cytokines [40,13,41]; inhibition of antimicrobial peptide production by Th2 cytokines [42]; upregulation of S100As by IL-17 and IL-22 [36]; and induction of epidermal hyperplasia by IL-22 [36]. Interestingly, proinflammatory factors including cytokines (e.g. TSLP, type 2 cytokines and cytokine IL-31) and secreted molecules (e.g. histamine) – which are all present in inflamed eczematous skin – can also affect cutaneous somatosensory nerves directly and via the release of pruritogens [43]. Such crosstalk between the immune and nervous systems is poorly understood, but may contribute to the severe itch of atopic eczema. This causes the patient considerable discomfort and provokes repetitive scratching, which can subsequently alter peripheral and central neural sensitisation to provoke further pruritus – the 'itch-scratch cycle' [44]. This chronic scratching results in further damage to the skin barrier.

Atopic eczema is associated with systemic immune effects, including skewing of the immune system towards Th2-type responses. As previously discussed, neonatal atopic eczema is associated with other chronic atopic conditions, including asthma (which is in part mediated by activated Th2 lymphocytes in the respiratory epithelia) and sensitisation to food allergens. In many individuals, atopic eczema is associated with high levels of circulating specific and nonspecific IgE, with associated immediate type allergies. IgE can result in direct activation of mast cells and certain skin-resident antigen presenting cells (e.g Langerhans' cells) via high affinity *FcεR1* receptors [45]. However, the precise role of IgE in cutaneous inflammation is not clear, with more recent aetiological studies focusing on the T cell infiltrate. The production of allergen-specific IgE is seen in murine models of atopic eczema, such as following the topical application of ovalbumin in 'flaky tail' mice, with the concurrent development of Th2-type cutaneous inflammation [28]. However, it is possible that IgE formation is primarily an epiphenomenon or even a downstream consequence of severe skin inflammation [46].

MICROBIOME

The skin represents the interface between our immune system and the microbial world, which is an important factor in the aetiopathogenesis of atopic eczema.

The skin microbiota refers to the global array of micro-organisms (including bacteria, fungi and viruses) living in the skin microenvironment, which is regionally defined by differing sebum, moisture content (sweat), skin pH and hair follicle density. We know that the skin microbiome is dysregulated in atopic eczema, in particular with overgrowth of the bacterium *S. aureus*. However, with the advent of pyrosequencing technology, which is able to identify around 80% more bacterial strains than conventional culture-based methods, much greater complexity and diversity of skin microbiota has been demonstrated [47,48]. Healthy skin is colonised by highly diverse bacterial communities composed of hundreds of different species. However, the most abundant taxa stably present are *Propionibacteria*, *Staphylococcus* and *Corynebacterium*. Abundances vary between dry, moist and sebaceous body sites, but remain surprisingly stable within these ecological niches throughout life [47, 48]. Using similar approaches, it has also been demonstrated that there are diverse communities of skin fungi. Strikingly, the microbiome even extends into subepidermal compartments of normal skin, with bacterial 16S rRNA detected within the dermis and dermal adipose tissue [49]. In addition, the interplay between skin commensals and the skin immune system appears important in aiding the development of a regulatory T cell, cytokine and complement network in the skin [50]. Skin commensals such as *Staphylococcus epidermidis* modulate local T cells through the tuning of cytokines such as IL-1, and it is likely that microbial metabolites are recognised by epidermal antigen-presenting cells [50]. The presence of microbial metabolites within the dermis may also contribute to the crosstalk between commensals, potential pathogens and the skin immune system.

In established atopic eczema the skin is in a state of dysbiosis, with significant changes seen in the composition of the bacterial microbiome. Numerous culture-based studies support the clinical link between *S. aureus* burden and eczema severity [51,52]. Greater skin barrier disruption, as measured by TEWL, is correlated with greater *S. aureus* colonisation [53]. In addition, staphylococcal peptides and their super-antigens have also been implicated in driving eczematous inflammation – for instance, staphylococcal delta toxin can lead to mast cell degranulation whilst alpha toxin induces keratinocyte apoptosis; T cells are stimulated by staphylococcal enterotoxins that can act as superantigens; and certain staphylococcal surface proteins can modulate inflammation (e.g. protein A) [54–57]. In addition, *S. aureus* can drive eczematous inflammation in animal models [58]. More recently, sequencing of skin microbiota from children with atopic eczema has demonstrated that *S. epidermidis* may also be involved in disease pathogenesis [59]. Atopic eczema flares were not only associated with a significant fall in skin microbiota diversity, but also a parallel increase in abundance of both *S. aureus* and *S. epidermidis*. Of note, topical anti-inflammatory and antimicrobial treatment immediately following the flare was associated with reduced abundance of *S. aureus* and a restoration of diversity.

Despite the clear association between the bacterial microbiome and atopic eczema (through the use of novel 16sRNA sequencing technology), it remains uncertain whether bacterial dysbiosis of the skin plays a causal role in the development of atopic eczema and disease flares, or whether the observed expansion of *S. aureus* and reduction in bacterial diversity are primarily an epiphenomenon resulting from an impaired and inflamed skin barrier. Thus, a better understanding of the complex interplay between the immune system, microbiome and skin barrier may lead to novel therapeutic strategies, such as the topical application of probiotics that enhance cutaneous microbial diversity.

THERAPEUTICS

The key to successful long-term management of atopic eczema involves maintaining and repairing the skin barrier with emollients, reducing inflammation with topical or systemic immunosuppressants, and eliminating any exacerbating factors – such as infection, allergens and irritants. Patients should be fully involved in their own care, and should be able to access psychological support if needed. This multistep approach to the management of atopic eczema in adults and children is outlined in national and international guidelines [60–65].

The regular application of emollients to the skin is central to the treatment of atopic eczema. This delivers lipids to the epidermis to help restore barrier homeostasis, which in turn can reduce disease severity, symptoms and the need for topical corticosteroids [66]. Novel emollient preparations have also been developed that contain specific components of the epidermal barrier, such as ceramides and essential fatty acids; however, these do not have clear superiority over conventional emollients. To limit potential irritation and/or sensitisation, patients should stick to products without unnecessary ingredients, such as fragrances.

Topical treatments that target skin inflammation in atopic eczema include corticosteroids and calcineurin inhibitors. In acute atopic eczema, patients should be advised to use an appropriate strength topical corticosteroid for the body site affected at least once daily, with treatment reviewed regularly and tailored accordingly [67]. It is well established that prolonged use of topical corticosteroids can result in side effects, including skin atrophy, as well as systemic absorption. Topical calcineurin inhibitors offer an alternative to corticosteroids – pimecrolimus 1% cream is licensed in the UK for mild-to-moderate atopic eczema, and is often used to treat the face and neck in children aged ≥2 years old; tacrolimus 0.1% ointment is more effective than pimecrolimus [68], is licensed in the UK for moderate-to-severe atopic eczema, and can be used in patients 16 years and older (0.03%, ≥2 years). In addition to treating acute atopic eczema, topical corticosteroids and calcineurin inhibitors both have a role in maintaining disease remission, with twice weekly application to troublesome sites shown to prophylactically reduce disease flares [69].

Second and third-line treatments for moderate-to-severe atopic eczema include UV phototherapy and systemic immunomodulatory medications such as corticosteroids (for acute flares), ciclosporin, azathioprine, methotrexate and mycophenolate mofetil. Narrow-band UVB and medium-dose UVA1 are the preferred phototherapy modalities; however, phototherapy is not universally effective, and is associated with a cumulative risk of skin cancer [70]. Although several different systemic agents are used, an 8-week course of oral ciclosporin is the only oral medication licensed for adults with chronic atopic eczema. Much of the clinical evidence for these agents is based on small and heterogeneous studies, with little comparative data. Ciclosporin seems to work most rapidly, reducing disease severity by about 50% following 6–8 weeks of treatment. However, patients often re-flare quickly upon stopping treatment [71]. The full clinical effect of both azathioprine and methotrexate takes longer to declare itself (often up to 3 months), but these agents potentially alter the disease natural history in the long-term [72]. It is important to note that systemic treatments for atopic eczema have different side effect profiles, different contraindications, and largely require regular blood test monitoring throughout treatment. Therefore, the choice of agent should ultimately be tailored to the patient.

Meta-analyses of the routine use of antibacterial treatments in atopic eczema have shown no clear benefit [73], and such approaches risk facilitating the development of microbial resistance. Therefore, the use of topical and systemic antibiotics is recommended only where there is clear clinical evidence of secondary bacterial infection. However, a recent randomised controlled trial (RCT) in children showed that regular dilute bleach baths, in combination with nasal bacterial decolonisation, can reduce disease severity [74].

Current conventional systemic treatments for atopic eczema have limited efficacy and potential toxic side effects. As a result, uncontrolled atopic eczema represents a considerable burden and unmet need. Our increasing understanding of disease pathogenesis has led to the development of novel targeted therapeutic strategies, such as biologic agents.

As already outlined, lymphocyte activation is central to the inflammation seen in atopic eczema, and key to this are Th2 cells and other lymphocyte subsets producing the type 2 cytokines IL-4, IL-5 and IL-13. Selective antagonists targeting these proinflammatory mediators, such as monoclonal antibodies (mAb), represent promising new therapeutic agents. Establishing this approach is dupilumab, a monoclonal antibody (mAb) that binds to and blocks the common alpha chain of the IL-4 receptor (IL-4Rα), blocking the actions of IL-4 and IL-13. A recent Phase 2b RCT in moderate-to-severe atopic eczema showed a major improvement in disease activity of 68–74% (high dose dupilumab groups) at 16 weeks, compared with 18% in the placebo group [75]. In addition, dupilimab treatment was associated with both reduced epidermal hyperplasia and an improvement in molecular markers of disease activity. Notably, there was also a transition in the mRNA transcriptome of involved skin towards that of nonlesional skin [76]. These findings confirm the importance of Th2-like inflammation in atopic eczema. Mepolizumab is a mAb against the type 2 cytokine IL-5, which is important in eosinophil recruitment and proliferation. Despite efficacy in asthma, this biologic only led to a moderate improvement in patients with atopic eczema [77], although a reduction in peripheral eosinophilia was noted. These data may indicate that IL-5 is less important to the pathogenesis of atopic eczema. Several other mAb molecular targets are under investigation but currently unreported, including IL-13 (tralokinumab, lebrikizumab), TSLP (AMG157), and the pruritus-associated cytokine IL-31 (CIM331).

As outlined above, the majority of patients with atopic eczema develop IgE antibodies to common environmental allergens. Omalizumab, a mAb against IgE, is effective in patients with asthma and chronic spontaneous urticaria; however, it is not clearly effective in chronic atopic eczema, despite abrogating acute allergic responses [78]. This, together with the observation that dupilumab appears to be effective irrespective of IgE status, suggests that the development of allergen-specific IgE is not a key driver of the cutaneous inflammation seen in atopic eczema. Nevertheless, other novel methods to deplete circulating IgE in patients with atopic eczema are currently under investigation, including IgE immunoadsorption [79].

Small molecule antagonists represent another therapeutic strategy for atopic eczema. These include topical and oral PDE4 inhibitors, with preliminary data showing that the oral agent apremilast may have similar efficacy to conventional systemic immunosuppressants already in use, such as ciclosporin [80]. It is also possible that janus kinase inhibitors, which specifically block cytokine signaling pathways and are increasingly used in other chronic inflammatory conditions, have a potential role in the management of atopic eczema.

Many novel treatment approaches are currently focused on downstream immunological targets. However, given that the defective epidermal barrier is a common precursor to disease, a focus on repairing this may prove to be a powerful and complementary therapeutic strategy. Indeed, experiments on 'flaky tail' mice (which have a *FLG* null mutation) and human skin equivalents in vitro have shown that it is possible to restore key barrier components such as filaggrin, which in mice was found to improve histological features of diseased skin [81]. In addition to treating the condition, such approaches may even prevent the development of atopic eczema in high-risk groups.

PREVENTION

Strategies to prevent atopic eczema altogether are attracting increasing interest. The most promising approach thus far aims to use 'barrier therapy' in early life to prevent the initiation and progression of the condition. Two small independent studies have reported encouraging data, although larger trials are needed. In a RCT of 124 high-risk neonates, parents in the intervention arm applied full-body emollient therapy at least once daily, starting within 3 weeks of birth. Parents in the control arm were asked to use no emollients. The authors reported a 50% relative risk reduction on cumulative atopic eczema incidence at 6 months in the emollient group [82]. A similar Japanese study including high-risk 118 neonates found that those receiving daily emollients had a significantly lower risk of developing atopic eczema by 32 weeks compared to control subjects. However, there was no effect on egg sensitisation as measured by specific IgE [83]. Evidence for the utility of emollients as a preventative strategy will be extended by a large-scale RCT in which around 1300 participants will be randomised to daily emollients for a year, or standard skin care advice only [(BEEP) – barrier enhancement for eczema prevention].

With atopic eczema historically classified as an allergic disease, until recently there has been a focus on allergen avoidance [84]. However, overall results have been inconsistent or disappointing. A 2012 Cochrane review combined data from two studies (334 pregnant women), finding no protective effect of maternal dietary antigen avoidance during pregnancy or lactation on the incidence of atopic eczema during the first 18 months of life [85]. Of note, the restricted diet during pregnancy was associated with a slight but significantly lower mean gestational weight gain, a nonsignificant increase in risk of preterm birth, and a nonsignificant reduction in mean birth weight.

The same authors wrote a second Cochrane review analysing the impact of exclusive breastfeeding on several atopic outcomes. Two large observational studies conducted in two different countries were pooled to provide data on atopic eczema, with the conclusion that exclusive breastfeeding for 6–7 months conferred no protection against developing atopic eczema at 5–7 years compared with exclusive breastfeeding for 3–4 months [86].

Nutritional supplements have also been investigated as an approach to prevent atopic eczema. For instance, probiotics are viable micro-organisms (such as lactobacilli and bifidobacteria) that may exert beneficial health effects on the host, whereas prebiotics are nondigestible carbohydrates that stimulate the growth of probiotic bacteria in the gut. These have been used alone or in combination in an attempt to prevent allergic disease, with the rationale that lack of microbial exposure or diversity during infancy and early childhood may shift the Th1/Th2 cytokine balance towards an allergic Th2 response and increased atopic eczema risk. There have been six systematic reviews analysing the effectiveness of this strategy for preventing atopic eczema, with varying results. However, the best evidence suggests that probiotics can safely reduce the risk of atopic eczema by up to 50%, with lactobacillus strains appearing most effective. The WAO guidelines [87] now recommend probiotics in women during pregnancy and breastfeeding, but they remain vague on the optimal delivery protocol, including timing (prenatal, postnatal or both), recipients (mother, baby or both), and whether single or mixed bacterial strains should be used.

Other research on nutritional supplements has looked at the role of maternal vitamin D intake on atopic eczema risk in the child. One review found three relevant studies, although data was not pooled. Two of these (2109 participants total) found no link, but the third study of 763 mothers and children reported that vitamin D intake of >172 IU/day during pregnancy was associated with a 37% reduction in the odds of parent-reported atopic eczema in children aged 6–24 months [88].

Finally, preliminary evidence that water hardness may increase the risk of developing atopic eczema [27] raises the question of whether installing water softeners around the time of birth can prevent the condition developing in infants. This is an area of active current research.

CONCLUSION

We have reviewed recent advances in the field of atopic eczema, focusing first on how diverse inherited and acquired abnormalities in epidermal structural and enzymatic proteins converge to impair skin barrier function and result in increased susceptibility to atopic eczema. We have also explored the impact of the defective skin barrier on immune responses and the skin microbiome. Although the primary pathogenic events in atopic eczema are not known, there is a complex interplay between the epidermal barrier and host immune activation, which in turn determines the response to environmental factors, such as allergens and microbes. Ongoing research to characterise this relationship further will lead to a new era of combined management, aiming to simultaneously address both the epidermal susceptibility and cutaneous inflammation. For now, the identification of effective biologics in eczema is at last heralding real progress in developing an armamentarium to rival that enjoyed by patients with psoriasis for the past decade. Finally, the emerging 'outside-in' paradigm of atopic eczema is driving research into the prevention of atopic eczema – and indeed other atopic conditions – via early 'barrier therapy' that may also minimise early transcutaneous allergic sensitisation. Thus, understanding the pathogenesis of atopic eczema has implications far beyond treatment and prevention of the disease itself, as it may also hold the key to halting the progression to food and respiratory allergies.

Key points for clinical practice

- Atopic eczema is a common and highly debilitating chronic inflammatory skin disorder.
- Immune dysregulation plays a key role, but recent evidence has shifted the focus to disruption of the skin barrier as the key precursor.
- Loss-of-function mutations in the *FLG* gene are the strongest known genetic risk factor, but there are numerous environmental and immunological factors that influence both the disease manifestation and its course.
- The current therapeutic armamentarium is largely limited to simple barrier-enhancing emollients, topical anti-inflammatory agents, and systemic immunosuppressive therapies. However, there are several emerging therapies that include targeted biologics and small molecule compounds.
- Increased recognition of the 'outside-in' paradigm of atopic eczema is driving research into preventative strategies for atopic eczema and other atopic conditions.

REFERENCES

1. Flohr C, Mann J. New insights into the epidemiology of childhood atopic dermatitis. Allergy 2014; 69:3–16.
2. Beattie P, Lewis-Jones M. A comparative study of impairment of quality of life in children with skin disease and children with other chronic childhood diseases. Br J Dermatol 2006; 155:145–151.
3. Herd RM, Tidman MJ, Prescott RJ, Hunter JA. The cost of atopic eczema. Br J Dermatol 1996; 135:20–23.
4. Mancini AJ, Kaulback K, Chamlin SL. The socioeconomic impact of atopic dermatitis in the United States: a systematic review. Pediatr Dermatol 2008; 25:1–6.
5. Paternoster L, Standl M, Waage J, et al. Multi-ancestry genome-wide association study of 21,000 cases and 95,000 controls identifies new risk loci for atopic dermatitis. Nat Genet 2015; 47:1449–1456.
6. Hanifin JM, Rajika G. Diagnostic features of atopic dermatitis. Acta Dermato-Venereologica 1980; 92:44–47.
7. Williams HC, Burney PG, Hay RJ, et al. The U.K. Working Party's Diagnostic Criteria for Atopic Dermatitis. I. Derivation of a minimum set of discriminators for atopic dermatitis. Br J Dermatol 1994; 131:383–396.
8. Cork MJ, Robinson DA, Vasilopoulos Y, et al. New perspectives on epidermal barrier dysfunction in atopic dermatitis: gene-environment interactions. J Allergy Clin Immunol 2006; 118:3–21.
9. Palmer CN, Irvine AD, Terron-Kwiatkowski A, et al. Common loss-of-function variants of the epidermal barrier protein filaggrin are a major predisposing factor for atopic dermatitis. Nat Genet 2006; 38:441–446.
10. Weidinger S, Novak N. Atopic dermatitis. Lancet 2016; 387:1109–1122.
11. Tsakok T, Flohr C. Filaggrin and atopic dermatitis (Chapter 16). Thyssen & Maibach's Filaggrin Molecules in Health and Disease. Springer USA 2014.
12. Weidinger S1, O'Sullivan M, Illig T, et al. Filaggrin mutations, atopic eczema, hay fever, and asthma in children. J Allergy Clin Immunol 200; 121:1203–1209e1.
13. Howell MD, Kim BE, Gao P, et al. Cytokine modulation of atopic dermatitis filaggrin skin expression. J Allergy Clin Immunol 2007; 120:150–155.
14. Brown SJ, Kroboth K, Sandilands A, et al. Intragenic copy number variation within filaggrin contributes to the risk of atopic dermatitis with a dose-dependent effect. J Invest Dermatol 2012; 132:98–104.
15. Morar N, Cookson WO, Harper JI, Moffatt MF. Filaggrin mutations in children with severe atopic dermatitis. J Invest Dermatol 2007; 127:1667–1672.
16. Pellerin L, Henry J, Hsu CY, et al. Defects of filaggrin-like proteins in both lesional and nonlesional atopic skin. J Allergy Clin Immunol 2013; 131:1094–102.
17. De Benedetto A, Rafaels NM, McGirt LY, et al. Tight junction defects in patients with atopic dermatitis. J Allergy Clin Immunol 2011; 127:773–786.e1–7.
18. De Benedetto A, Slifka MK, Rafaels NM, et al. Reductions in claudin-1 may enhance susceptibility to herpes simplex virus 1 infections in atopic dermatitis. J Allergy Clin Immunol 2011; 128:242–246.e5.
19. Tsakok T, Marrs T, Mohsin M, et al. Does atopic dermatitis cause food allergy? A systematic review. J Allergy Clin Immunol 2016; 137:1071–1078.
20. Lack G, Fox D, Northstone K, Golding J. Avon Longitudinal Study of Parents and Children Study Team. Factors associated with the development of peanut allergy in childhood. N Engl J Med 2003; 348:977–985.
21. Brown SJ, Asai Y, Cordell HJ, et al. Loss-of-function variants in the filaggrin gene are a significant risk factor for peanut allergy. J Allergy Clin Immunol 2011; 127:661–667.
22. Brough HA, Liu AH, Sicherer S, et al. Atopic dermatitis increases the effect of exposure to peanut antigen in dust on peanut sensitization and likely peanut allergy. J Allergy Clin Immunol 2015; 135:164–670.
23. Flohr C, Perkin M, Logan K, et al. Atopic dermatitis and disease severity are the main risk factors for food sensitization in exclusively breastfed infants. J Invest Dermatol 2014; 134:345–350.
24. Cardona ID, Stillman L, Jain N. Does bathing frequency matter in pediatric atopic dermatitis? Ann Allergy Asthma Immunol 2016; 117:9–13.
25. Sherriff A, Golding J; Alspac Study Team. Hygiene levels in a contemporary population cohort are associated with wheezing and atopic eczema in preschool infants. Arch Dis Child 2002; 87:26–29.
26. Silverberg JI, Hanifin J, Simpson EL. Climatic factors are associated with childhood eczema prevalence in the United States. J Invest Dermatol 2013; 133:1752–1759.
27. Perkin MR, Craven J, Logan K, et al. Association between domestic water hardness, chlorine, and atopic dermatitis risk in early life: A population-based cross-sectional study. J Allergy Clin Immunol 2016; pii: S0091-6749:30187–30187.
28. Fallon PG, Sasaki T, Sandilands A, et al. A homozygous frameshift mutation in the mouse FLG gene facilitates enhanced percutaneous allergen priming. Nat Genet 2009; 41:602–608.

29. Kezic S, O'Regan GM, Lutter R, et al. Filaggrin loss-of-function mutations are associated with enhanced expression of IL-1 cytokines in the stratum corneum of patients with atopic dermatitis and in a murine model of filaggrin deficiency. J Allergy Clin Immunol 2012; 129:1031–1039.

30. Scharschmidt TC, Man MQ, Hatano Y, et al. Filaggrin deficiency confers a paracellular barrier abnormality that reduces inflammatory thresholds to irritants and haptens. J Allergy Clin Immunol 2009; 124:496–506.

31. Dickel H, Gambichler T, Kamphowe J, Altmeyer P, Skrygan M. Standardized tape stripping prior to patch testing induces upregulation of Hsp90, Hsp70, IL-33, TNF-α and IL-8/CXCL8 mRNA: new insights into the involvement of 'alarmins'. Contact Dermatitis 2010; 63:215–222.

32. Leyva-Castillo JM, Hener P, Michea P, et al. Skin thymic stromal lymphopoietin initiates Th2 responses through an orchestrated immune cascade. Nat Commun 2013; 4:2847.

33. Black AP, Ardern-Jones MR, Kasprowicz V, et al. Human keratinocyte induction of rapid effector function in antigen-specific memory CD4+ and CD8+ T cells. Eur J Immunol 2007; 37:1485–1493.

34. Jarrett R, Salio M, Lloyd-Lavery A, et al. Filaggrin inhibits generation of CD1a neolipid antigens by house dust mite-derived phospholipase. Sci Transl Med 2016; 8:325ra18.

35. Suarez-Farinas M, Tintle SJ, Shemer A, et al. Nonlesional atopic dermatitis skin is characterized by broad terminal differentiation defects and variable immune abnormalities. J Allergy Clin Immunol 2011; 127:954–964.

36. Gittler JK, Shemer A, Suárez-Fariñas M, et al. Progressive activation of T(H)2/T(H)22 cytokines and selective epidermal proteins characterizes acute and chronic atopic dermatitis. J Allergy Clin Immunol 2012; 130:1344–1354.

37. Hijnen D, Knol EF, Gent YY, et al. CD8(+) T cells in the lesional skin of atopic dermatitis and psoriasis patients are an important source of IFN-γ, IL-13, IL-17, and IL-22. J Invest Dermatol 2013; 133:973–979.

38. Salimi M, Barlow JL, Saunders SP, et al. A role for IL-25 and IL-33-driven type-2 innate lymphoid cells in atopic dermatitis. J Exp Med 2013; 210:2939–2950.

39. Glatz M, Bosshard PP, Hoetzenecker W, Schmid-Grendelmeier P. The Role of Malassezia spp. in Atopic Dermatitis. J Clin Med 2015; 4:1217–1228.

40. Gutowska-Owsiak D, Schaupp AL, Salimi M, Taylor S, Ogg GS. Interleukin-22 downregulates filaggrin expression and affects expression of profilaggrin processing enzymes. Br J Dermatol 2011; 165:492–498.

41. Kim BE, Leung DY, Boguniewicz M, Howell MD. Loricrin and involucrin expression is down-regulated by Th2 cytokines through STAT-6. Clin Immunol 2008; 126:332–337.

42. Kopfnagel V, Harder J, Werfel T. Expression of antimicrobial peptides in atopic dermatitis and possible immunoregulatory functions. Curr Opin Allergy Clin Immunol 2013; 13:531–536.

43. Sonkoly E, Muller A, Lauerma AI, et al. IL-31: a new link between T cells and pruritus in atopic skin inflammation. J Allergy Clin Immunol 2006; 117:411–417.

44. Mollanazar NK, Smith PK, Yosipovitch G. Mediators of Chronic Pruritus in Atopic Dermatitis: Getting the Itch Out? Clin Rev Allergy Immunol 2016; 51:263–292.

45. Novak N. An update on the role of human dendritic cells in patients with atopic dermatitis. J Allergy Clin Immunol 2012; 129:879–886.

46. Strid J, Sobolev O, Zafirova B, Polic B, Hayday A. The intraepithelial T cell response to NKG2D-ligands links lymphoid stress surveillance to atopy. Science 2011; 334:1293–1297.

47. Costello EK, Lauber CL, Hamady M, et al. Bacterial community variation in human body habitats across space and time. Science 2009; 326:1694–1697.

48. Grice EA, Kong HH, Conlan S, et al. Topographical and temporal diversity of the human skin microbiome. Science 2009; 324:1190–1192.

49. Nakatsuji T, Chiang HI, Jiang SB, et al. The microbiome extends to subepidermal compartments of normal skin. Nat Commun 2013; 4:1431.

50. Belkaid Y, Segre JA. Dialogue between skin microbiota and immunity. Science 2014; 346:954–959.

51. Gong JQ, Lin L, Lin T, et al. Skin colonization by Staphylococcus aureus in patients with eczema and atopic dermatitis and relevant combined topical therapy: a double-blind multicentre randomized controlled trial. Br J Dermatol 2006; 155:680–687.

52. Leyden JJ, Marples RR, Kligman AM. Staphylococcus aureus in the lesions of atopic dermatitis. Br J Dermatol 1974; 90:525–530.

53. Jinnestal CL, Belfrage E, Bäck O, Schmidtchen A, Sonesson A. Skin barrier impairment correlates with cutaneous Staphylococcus aureus colonization and sensitization to skin-associated microbial antigens in adult patients with atopic dermatitis. Int J Dermatol 2014; 53:27–33.

54. Brauweiler AM, Goleva E, Leung DY. Th2 cytokines increase *Staphylococcus aureus* alpha toxin-induced keratinocyte death through the signal transducer and activator of transcription 6 (STAT6). J Invest Dermatol 2014; 134:2114–2121.

55. Ezepchuk YV, Leung DY, Middleton MH, et al. Staphylococcal toxins and protein A differentially induce cytotoxicity and release of tumor necrosis factor-alpha from human keratinocytes. J Invest Dermatol 1996; 107:603–609.

56. Nakamura Y, Oscherwitz J, Cease KB, et al. Staphylococcus δ-toxin induces allergic skin disease by activating mast cells. Nature 2013; 503:397–401.

57. Zollner TM, Wichelhaus TA, Hartung A, et al. Colonization with superantigen-producing *Staphylococcus aureus* is associated with increased severity of atopic dermatitis. Clin Exp Allergy. 2000; 30:994–1000.

58. Kobayashi T, Glatz M, Horiuchi K, et al. Dysbiosis and *Staphylococcus aureus* Colonization Drives Inflammation in Atopic Dermatitis. Immunity 2015; 42:756–766.

59. Kong HH, Oh J, Deming C, et al. Temporal shifts in the skin microbiome associated with disease flares and treatment in children with atopic dermatitis. Genome Res 2012; 22:850–859.

60. Eichenfield LF, Tom WL, Berger TG, et al. Guidelines of care for the management of atopic dermatitis: section 2. Management and treatment of atopic dermatitis with topical therapies. J Am Acad Dermatol 2014; 71:116–132.

61. National Institute for Health and Clinical Excellence (NICE). Atopic eczema in under 12s: diagnosis and management [CG57]. Published 2007. Accessed 2016.

62. Ring J, Alomar A, Bieber T, et al. Guidelines for treatment of atopic eczema (atopic dermatitis) part I. J Eur Acad Dermatol Venereol 2012; 26:1045–1060.

63. Ring J, Alomar A, Bieber T, et al. Guidelines for treatment of atopic eczema (atopic dermatitis) Part II. J Eur Acad Dermatol Venereol 2012; 26:1176–1193.

64. Sidbury R, Davis DM, Cohen DE, et al. Guidelines of care for the management of atopic dermatitis: section 3. Management and treatment with phototherapy and systemic agents. J Am Acad Dermatol 2014; 71:327–349.

65. Sidbury R, Tom WL, Bergman JN, et al. Guidelines of care for the management of atopic dermatitis: Section 4. Prevention of disease flares and use of adjunctive therapies and approaches. J Am Acad Dermatol 2014; 71:1218–1233.

66. Lindh JD, Bradley M. Clinical Effectiveness of Moisturizers in Atopic Dermatitis and Related Disorders: A Systematic Review. Am J Clin Dermatol 2015; 16:341–359.

67. Hoare C, Li Wan Po A, Williams H. Systematic review of treatments for atopic eczema. Health Technol Assess 2000; 4:1–191.

68. Paller AS, Lebwohl M, Fleischer AB Jr, et al. Tacrolimus ointment is more effective than pimecrolimus cream with a similar safety profile in the treatment of atopic dermatitis: results from 3 randomized, comparative studies. J Am Acad Dermatol 2005; 52:810–822.

69. Schmitt J, von Kobyletzki L, Svensson A, Apfelbacher C. Efficacy and tolerability of proactive treatment with topical corticosteroids and calcineurin inhibitors for atopic eczema: systematic review and meta-analysis of randomized controlled trials. Br J Dermatol 2011; 164:415–428.

70. Garritsen FM, Brouwer MW, Limpens J, Spuls PI. Photo(chemo)therapy in the management of atopic dermatitis: an updated systematic review with implications for practice and research. Br J Dermatol 2014; 170:501–5013.

71. Schmitt J, Schmitt N, Meurer M. Cyclosporin in the treatment of patients with atopic eczema – a systematic review and meta-analysis. J Eur Acad Dermatol Venereol 2007; 21:606–619.

72. Schram ME, Roekevisch E, Leeflang MM, et al. A randomized trial of methotrexate versus azathioprine for severe atopic eczema. J Allergy Clin Immunol 2011; 128:353–359.

73. Birnie AJ, Bath-Hextall FJ, Ravenscroft JC, Williams HC. Interventions to reduce *Staphylococcus aureus* in the management of atopic eczema. Cochrane Database Syst Rev 2008:CD003871.

74. Huang JT, Abrams M, Tlougan B, Rademaker A, Paller AS. Treatment of *Staphylococcus aureus* colonization in atopic dermatitis decreases disease severity. Pediatrics 2009; 123:e808–814.

75. Thaçi D, Simpson EL, Beck LA, et al. Efficacy and safety of dupilumab in adults with moderate-to-severe atopic dermatitis inadequately controlled by topical treatments: a randomised, placebo-controlled, dose-ranging phase 2b trial. Lancet 2016; 387:40–52.

76. Beck LA, Thaçi D, Hamilton JD, et al. Dupilumab treatment in adults with moderate-to-severe atopic dermatitis. N Engl J Med 2014; 371:130–139.

77. Oldhoff JM, Darsow U, Werfel T, et al. Anti-IL-5 recombinant humanized monoclonal antibody (mepolizumab) for the treatment of atopic dermatitis. Allergy 2005; 60:693–696.

78. Heil PM, Maurer D, Klein B, Hultsch T, Stingl G. Omalizumab therapy in atopic dermatitis: depletion of IgE does not improve the clinical course – a randomized, placebo-controlled and double blind pilot study. J Dtsch Dermatol Ges 2010; 8:990–998.

79. Kasperkiewicz M, Schmidt E, Frambach Y, et al. Improvement of treatment-refractory atopic dermatitis by immunoadsorption: a pilot study. J Allergy Clin Immunol 2011; 127:267–270.

80. Samrao A, Berry TM, Goreshi R, Simpson EL. A pilot study of an oral phosphodiesterase inhibitor (apremilast) for atopic dermatitis in adults. Arch Dermatol 2012; 148:890–897.

81. Stout TE, McFarland T, Mitchell JC, Appukuttan B, Stout JT. Recombinant filaggrin is internalized and processed to correct filaggrin deficiency. J Invest Dermatol 2014; 134:423–429.

82. Simpson EL, Chalmers JR, Hanifin JM, et al. Emollient enhancement of the skin barrier from birth offers effective atopic dermatitis prevention. J Allergy Clin Immunol 2014; 134:818–823.

83. Horimukai K, Morita K, Narita M, et al. Application of moisturizer to neonates prevents development of atopic dermatitis. J Allergy Clin Immunol 2014; 134:824–830.

84. Flohr C, Mann J. New approaches to the prevention of childhood atopic dermatitis. Allergy 2014; 69:56–61.

85. Kramer MS, Kakuma R. Maternal dietary antigen avoidance during pregnancy or lactation, or both, for preventing or treating atopic disease in the child. Cochrane Database Syst Rev 2012:CD000133.

86. Kramer MS, Kakuma R. Optimal duration of exclusive breastfeeding. Cochrane Database Syst Rev 2012:CD003517.

87. Fiocchi A, Pawankar R, Cuello-Garcia C, et al. World Allergy Organization-McMaster University Guidelines for Allergic Disease Prevention (GLAD-P): Probiotics. World Allergy Organ J 2015; 8:4.

88. Christesen HT, Elvander C, Lamont RF, Jørgensen JS. The impact of vitamin D in pregnancy on extraskeletal health in children: a systematic review. Acta Obstet Gynecol Scand 2012; 91:1368–1380.

Chapter 7

Benign and malignant penile lesions

Tang Ngee Shim, Asif Muneer

INTRODUCTION

Male genital skin diseases encompass a wide variety of skin lesions and rashes which are often limited to the genital area although they may also represent a more generalised skin disorder. Genital lesions can have an impact on the physical, psychological as well as the sexual health of men and can present to a range of subspecialists including dermatology, genitourinary medicine and urology. An accurate differential diagnosis is required in order to promptly diagnose the premalignant and malignant lesions to avoid a delay in appropriate treatment. Important factors which are apparent in patients presenting with penile cancer is the delay in the patient presenting to a clinician, a delay in making the correct diagnosis as well as referral to the wrong subspecialists.

CLINICAL EVALUATION

History

A full medical and sexual history should be taken focusing on the characteristics of the lesion as well as the impact on sexual function. Patients may be asymptomatic or describe itch, pain, dyspareunia, bleeding, scaling, splitting of foreskin, difficulty in retracting the foreskin or ulceration. The circumcision status, sexual practices, contraceptive methods, and any drug history (both topical treatment to the penis and systemic treatment) should be documented.

A personal and family history of atopy and psoriasis can help to diagnose genital lesions which are associated with more generalised skin complaints.

Examination

An examination of the genital and extragenital skin including the mucosal surfaces, hair and nails is mandatory.

Tang Ngee Shim MB BCh, MD, FRCP Edin Consultant Dermatologist, Dermatology Department, University Hospital Coventry and Warwickshire, UK.

Asif Muneer MD FRCS(Urol), Consultant Urological Surgeon and Andrologist, Department of Urology and should state: NIHR Biomedical Research Centre University College London Hospital; Associate Professor, Division of Surgery and Interventional Science, University College London, UK. Email: Asif.Muneer@nhs.net (for correspondence)

If a foreskin is present then this needs to be gently retracted such that the entire glans penis and inner prepuce are visualised together with the frenulum. Pathological phimosis may prevent full retraction of the prepuce but clinicians should still maintain a high index of suspicion for underlying lesions on the glans and especially the coronal sulcus as this is a common site for premalignant and malignant penile lesions.

Features that should be documented include the appearance and site of the lesion. The presence of circumcoronal adhesions should be noted as well as the appearance of the frenulum which may be thickened or completely lost secondary to long-standing inflammation such as lichen sclerosus (LSc).

Often inflammatory lesions are given a ubiquitous name such as balanitis or balanoposthitis. However, more accurately the term balanitis describes inflammation of the glans penis, whereas posthitis is inflammation limited to the prepuce. If both areas are affected, then the term balanoposthitis is used. Balanitis is uncommon in circumcised men [1]. In many cases, a dysfunctional foreskin is a causal or contributing factor [1,2].

Finally for suspected malignant lesions, the inguinal lymph nodes should be palpated as these are the first draining lymph nodes for primary penile cancer.

Benign genital lesions

Although a number of penile lesions may cause concern for both patients and nonspecialists, they may be nothing more than normal variants which often just require patient reassurance rather than surgical intervention which in itself may disrupt the penile contour.

NORMAL VARIANTS ON THE PENIS AND SCROTUM

Angiokeratoma

Angiokeratomas are small (2–5 mm), red, blue or purple papules. These can occur as solitary or multiple lesions affecting the scrotum, penile shaft, or glans (**Figure 7.1**). Angiokeratomas require reassurance and no specific treatment although electrocautery or

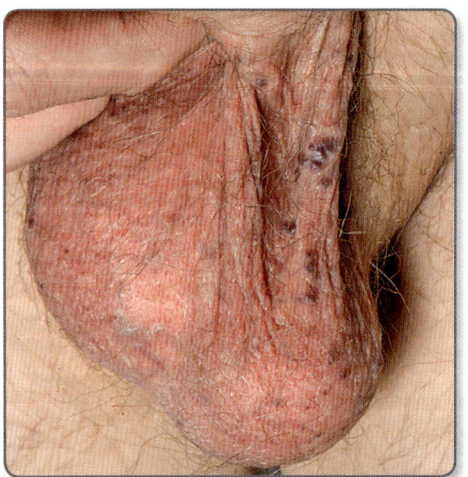

Figure 7.1 Angiokeratoma on the scrotum.

laser ablation can be used on lesions which are of concern to the patients due to cosmetic reasons. Anderson-Fabry disease, a rare inherited lysosomal storage disease, can present with multiple angiokeratomas in any region of the body, but are predominant around the abdomen and thighs.

Penile pearly papules

Penile pearly papules rarely involve the glans penis or penile shaft skin. These lesions present in two or three rows of uniform skin-coloured, smooth, rounded papules which are 1–2 mm in size, and located around the coronal margin or sulcus. Almost 50% of men have penile pearly papules and they can be mistaken for genital warts or ectopic sebaceous glands. Although asymptomatic, they can cause significant anxiety for men. Although they do not require any specific treatment, cryotherapy and laser treatment can be used to remove the lesions.

Sebaceous gland prominence

Sebaceous gland prominence, also known as Fox-Fordyce spots, sebaceous hyperplasia, and 'ectopic' sebaceous glands, are normal variants of the skin of the scrotal sac and penile shaft. Tyson glands are sebaceous glands present on the frenulum and on the coronal glans. Again patient reassurance should suffice.

Allergic and irritant contact dermatitis

Eczematous dermatoses affecting the genital skin in isolation are irritant contact dermatitis (ICD) and allergic contact dermatitis (ACD). There is an increased susceptibility of the genital skin to various allergens and irritants due to hygienic and sexual practices. ICD is concentration dependent (e.g. detergent) whereas ACD requires prior sensitisation (e.g. preservatives) [3]. Pain and burning (ICD), itch (ACD) and a persistent or recurrent erythematous scaly rash are the common presenting features. Genital ICD dermatitis is often due to over washing [4]. Other possible irritants include bodily fluids that may come into contact with this area (urine, sweat). Common allergens are found in lubricants, latex condoms, cleansing agents, disinfectants and treatments (corticosteroids, spermicides, antimicrobials, anaesthetics, preservatives or stabilisers) and perfumes or other contact agents transferred by hand. The most important aspects of management are the identification and avoidance of indictable irritants and allergens. The glans penis and foreskin may acquire contact dermatitis from products such as medicament used by a sexual partner so called connubial or consort allergic contact dermatitis. In both cases, it is essential to avoid the allergen or irritant and excessive washing. Soap substitutes, emollients, barrier protection and mild to moderate potency topical steroids can be used. Patch testing is the investigative tool in suspected ACD, particularly in cases unresponsive to treatment or a worsening of symptoms while topical treatments are being applied [3].

Seborrhoeic dermatitis

Seborrhoeic dermatitis is a common cause of balanoposthitis and may be associated with skin changes elsewhere (scalp, eyebrows, nasolabial folds, central chest, and upper back). It has both eczematous and psoriasiform features characterised by an erythematous patch with greasy yellowish scales. The exact aetiology is unknown although it may be due to an inherited or acquired hypersensitivity to commensal *Malassezia* yeast organisms [5]. Seborrhoeic dermatitis is common (up to 40%) in HIV and AIDS (up to 80%) compared with 3% of the normal population [6]. A Cochrane review reported several randomised control trials showing that topical corticosteroid treatment and azoles (such as ketoconazole and miconazole) are effective in reducing erythema, scaling and pruritus [6]. An antifungal shampoo such as ketoconazole 2% may be used as a soap substitute. There is also some benefit in using topical calcineurin inhibitors [7].

Psoriasis

Psoriasis is a common, chronic inflammatory disease of the skin affecting 1–8.5% of the adult population [8]. Symptoms include intense itching, pain and fissures but it may also be asymptomatic. The immunopathogenesis involves a complex genetically determined interplay between keratinocytes, dendritic cells and T cells [9]. However, isolated presentation of psoriasis on the genital skin is uncommon (2–5% of psoriatics) [10]. Affected areas include the pubic region, penis, skin folds and buttocks. It can often be part of the presentation of more generalised plaque psoriasis or inverse psoriasis, which involves skin folds or flexor surfaces such as the ears, axillae, groins, inframammary folds and the intergluteal crease, a phenotype that overlaps with seborrhoeic dermatitis. On the circumcised men, genital psoriasis presents with well-demarcated scaly erythematous patches of plaques. Scale is often absent on the glans or in the foreskin of the uncircumcised male. The Koebner phenomenon is common in the genital area because of the constant friction, exposure to irritants and occlusion.

Treatment with short-term mild to moderate topical corticosteroids is recommended [11]. If the response is unsatisfactory, or they require continuous treatment to maintain control and there is serious risk of steroid atrophy, topical calcineurin inhibitors can be initiated [11]. Low concentration tar preparations and topical vitamin D analogues also have a role. Systemic treatment may be considered for severe, recalcitrant cases of anogenital psoriasis [1,10].

Zoon's balanitis

Classical Zoon's plasma cell balanitis is a benign chronic irritation affecting middle-aged or elderly uncircumcised men. Clinically, the lesions are well-demarcated, shiny, symmetrical reddish (erythema) brown (hemosiderin) patches affecting the glans or foreskin. There is no involvement of the keratinised genital skin. Histologically, it is characterised by plasma cells in the dermal infiltrate. The important differential diagnosis is erythroplasia of Queyrat (EQ) – penile intraepithelial neoplasia (PeIN) limited to the glans penis or visceral foreskin. Although topical mild or potent topical corticosteroids can be helpful, circumcision is the definitive treatment [1,4].

Lichen sclerosus

Male genital LSc is a chronic acquired inflammatory skin disorder with a predilection for genital skin. There is a bimodal age incidence with peaks in young boys and in the fourth decade for adult men [12,13]. The symptomatology is rather diverse. Patients may be asymptomatic or describe itching, burning, bleeding, tearing, splitting, blisters, dyspareunia, difficulty retracting the foreskin or changes in the appearance of the genitalia (**Figure 7.2**) [1,12]. Meatal stenosis may lead to discomfort with urination, narrowing of the urinary stream and urinary obstruction; urethral stricture disease can be a severe

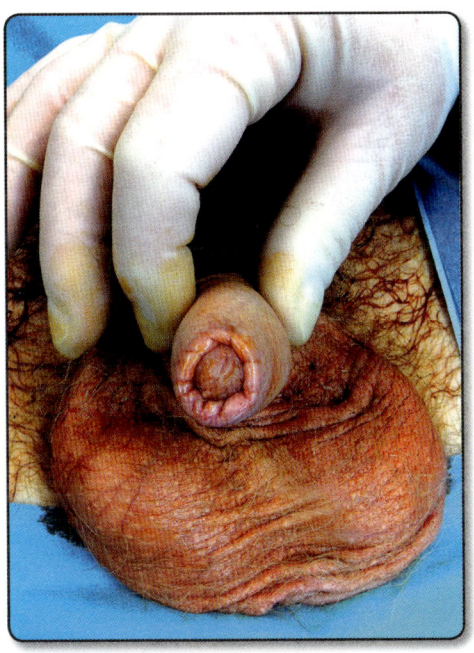

Figure 7.2 Early onset scarring on retracting the prepuce.

complication [14,15]. It is almost certainly due to chronic occluded exposure of susceptible epithelium to urine; most men confess to urinary dribbling/microincontinence [16]. The morphological features of LSc are similarly variable, including atrophic white patches or plaques on the glans and prepuce associated with zoonoid inflammation (**Figures 7.3** and **7.4**), lilac, slightly scaly patches (lichenoid inflammation) with telangeictasia and purpura, bullae and erosions and ulceration (**Figure 7.2**). Repeated chronic inflammation results in the formation of circumcoronal adhesions, scarring and effacement of the architecture. This can manifest as constrictive posthitis or even phimosis with the risk of urinary retention in severe cases. The diagnosis of genital LSc is made clinically. Biopsy should be considered if the clinical diagnosis is in doubt, or if recommended first line treatment fails after appropriate treatment duration or if malignancies are suspected. Typical histological features of LS are orthohyperkeratosis, epidermal atrophy, basal cell degeneration, dermal hyalinisation and a band like lymphocytic infiltrate. However, in early LSc, hyalinisation of the upper dermis may be lacking.

The aims of management are the restoration of normal sexual and urinary function. This may lead to a reduction of the risk of progression into the urethra and also the development of penile cancer. The association of genital LSc and squamous cell carcinoma (SCC) is widely recognised and the published risk ranges between 0% and 12.5% [12,17–21]. Initially one or two courses of ultrapotent topical corticosteroids under supervision can be used [12,22–24]. Topical calcineurin inhibitors have been advocated but the rationale is questionable and the safety equivocal, unlike the management strategy above which cures most patients and where no cancers have developed in years of follow-up [12,24]. All patients should be instructed to use emollients, and soap substitutes to minimise irritation of the genital skin.

Surgical intervention, commonly circumcision is indicated when topical corticosteroid therapy has failed, or phimosis, meatal stenosis, urethral stricture, PeIN and SCC is present.

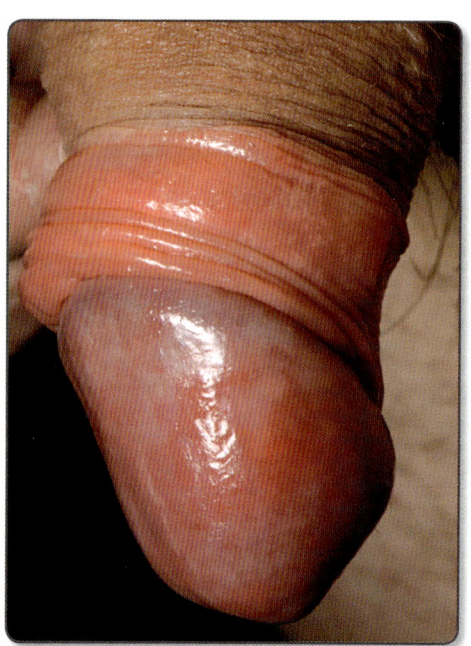

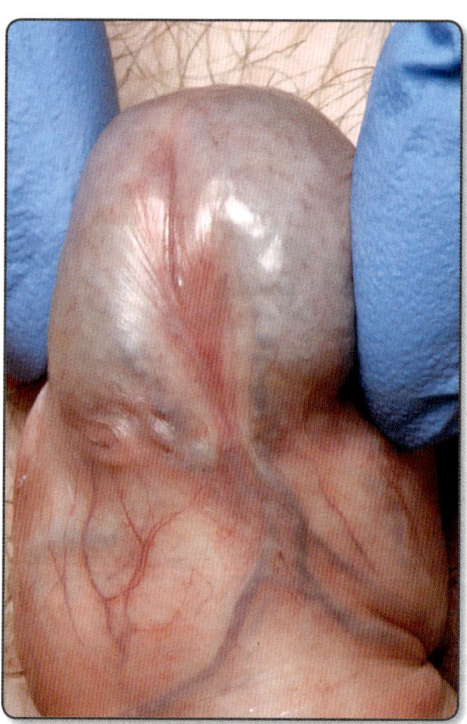

Figure 7.3 Zoonoid inflammation with lichenoid inflammation of the inner foreskin causing constrictive posthitis.

Figure 7.4 Effacement and loss of corona sulcus and frenulum.

Despite undergoing a circumcision, the glans can remain unresponsive to topical steroids in which case men are offered a glans resurfacing procedure [25].

Lichen planus

Lichen planus is a common inflammatory skin disease that can affect the skin, mucous membranes, hair follicles, and nails. The aetiology is thought to be a T-cell mediated autoimmune disease. Lichen planus is usually symptomatic, characterised by pain, burning, or itching and associated with dyspareunia. The primary lesions present as small, polygonal, violaceous, smooth flat-topped annular papules with a white reticulate surface (Wickham's striae, **Figure 7.5**) that resolve leaving postinflammatory hyperpigmentation. Mucosal lichen planus is a chronic condition with remissions and exacerbations, whereas cutaneous lesions tends to spontaneously resolve within a few years [26]. There is a predilection for the flexor wrists, torso, medial thighs, anterior shins, dorsum of the hands and the glans penis. Approximately 25% of men with cutaneous lichen planus have annular genital involvement [27]. The glans is the most common site for genital lichen planus probably reflecting the Koebner phenomenon. Biopsy may be necessary if the diagnosis is uncertain or more importantly, there is suspicion of PeIN or SCC. Characteristic histological findings include the presence of a band like intense lymphocytic inflammatory infiltrate in the dermis with basal layer degeneration and civatte bodies.

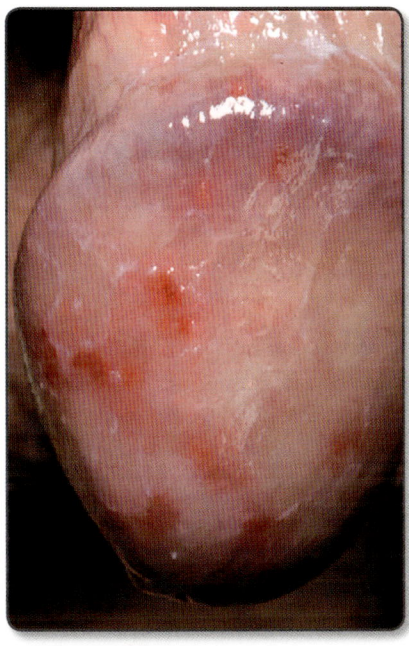

Figure 7.5 Wickham striae on the glans penis.

Potent or ultrapotent topical corticosteroids are the first-line treatment [4]. Circumcision is necessary for phimosis and should be considered in recalcitrant erosive disease [1]. Stubborn or widespread extragenital disease can be treated with systemic corticosteroids, retinoids (acitretin) or ciclosporin.

Nonspecific balanoposthitis

Nonspecific balanoposthitis is a manifestation of a dysfunctional foreskin. It is a diagnosis of exclusion and patients often present with dyspareunia. Clinical presentations can be variable, i.e. eczematous, psoriasiform, lichenoid or Zoonoid. However, histological biopsies tend to be nonspecific. Again circumcision is curative in most instances [1].

Warts

Genital warts are common in men. Most patients only complain of the presence of the lesions. Clinically, inapparent disease may present as balanoposthitis. The prevalence of human papillomavirus (HPV) in the genital tract of men is similar to that in women, and is between 3% and 45% depending on the age and population. The estimated lifetime risk of acquiring HPV sexually is between 50-80%. Congenital and acquired immunosuppression increases the susceptibility of the anogenital region to HPV infection and reactivation and progression to either dysplasia or invasive cancer. The clinical diagnosis of warts is usually certain, but the differential diagnosis includes condylomata lata, lichen planus, mollusca, Bowenoid papulosis (BP) and pearly penile papules. However, solitary lesions have a wider differential diagnosis, including giant condyloma and squamous cell carcinoma (SCC). Diagnostic biopsy is not necessary for typical genital warts. However, urgent biopsy or appropriate specialist referral must be considered if there is a clinical suspicion of neoplastic transformation, i.e. bleeding, irregular and unusual patterns of pigmentation, ulceration, or lesions with indurated dermal infiltration. Patients with anogenital warts and their partners may require a full sexually transmitted disease and sometimes colorectal assessment. Because evidence comparing efficacy is insufficient, the choice of treatment should depend on the person's preference, number, volume, type and site of lesions and the availability of treatment. The treatment generally involves topical agents (podophyllotoxin 0.15% cream or 0.5% solution, imiquimod 5% cream) or ablative treatment such as cryotherapy, excision and electrocautery [28,29].

Mollusca

Mollusca represent cutaneous infection with a human DNA poxvirus. Mollusca present as multiple, small, translucent dome-shaped papules with central 'umbilication' and are common in extragenital paediatric cases. Localised genital lesions are often seen in adults, perhaps in those who happened to avoid exposure or failed to acquire immunity during childhood. No treatment is required [30,31]. If patients opt for treatment, they must be informed that new lesions can appear for a while, necessitating more than one treatment course. No one treatment is advocated over another. In practice, podophyllotoxin 0.5%, imiquimod 5% cream, liquid nitrogen and curettage and cautery might be used [30,31].

Lichen nitidus

Lichen nitidus is a variant of lichen planus characterised by discrete and uniform, flat-topped itchy 1–2 mm micro papules. It is uncommon but usually seen as a widespread eruption in children. Whilst rarely affecting the genitals of adult men in isolation it can be confused with viral warts and Bowenoid Papulosis (BP) (an HPV-associated manifestation of PeIN).

Premalignant conditions of the penis

There are a number of premalignant penile lesions which are not related to HPV infection. These are primarily due to chronic inflammation, and include genital LSc, penile cutaneous horn, leukoplakia, and pseudoepitheliomatous, keratotic and micaceous balanitis. Unlike HPV-related tumours, progression of these premalignant lesions is largely into keratinising/verrucous SCC.

Premalignant lesions associated with high-risk HPV include Bowen's disease of the penis (BDP), Erythroplasia of Queyrat (EQ) and BP. 'High risk' HPV types 16 and 18 are the most common, and are found in 60–75% of PeIN and invasive tumors [31,32]. Low-risk HPV types 6 and 11 are associated with other premalignant lesions such as giant condylomata acuminata (GCA).

Penile intraepithelial neoplasia

Bowen's disease of the penis, BP and EQ are clinical expressions of squamous intraepithelial neoplasia. Histopathologically, these conditions are all the same in that they share identical features of squamous carcinoma in situ, i.e. acanthosis, parakeratotic or hyperkeratotic with full thickness epithelial dysplasia. Some authors have classified PeIN into grades I, II and III according to the degree of dysplasia on histological analysis [35]. The term PeIN is increasingly favoured to describe premalignant penile lesions. PeIN is further subclassified into differentiated, LS-associated and undifferentiated HPV-associated subtypes [36].

Erythroplasia of Queyrat affects the mucosal surfaces of the genitalia, such as the inner prepuce and glans, whereas BDP affects the keratinised skin of the penile shaft (**Figure 7.6**).

Lesions which occur in BDP are usually solitary, well defined, scaly, dull red plaques, often with areas of crusting. Occasionally, lesions may be heavily pigmented, resembling melanoma. While they primarily occur on the shaft, associated lesions are sometimes encountered in the inguinal and suprapubic region. Lesions may also occasionally have associated leukoplakic, nodular, or ulcerated changes.

Lesions in EQ are usually sharply defined plaques, which have a smooth, velvety, bright red appearance. They are usually painless, but can have areas of erosion. The vast majority occur in uncircumcised men with phimotic foreskins.

Invasive SCC has been reported in 5% of cases of BDP [37], while EQ has reported transformation rates of up to 30% [38,39].

Bowenoid papulosis

Unlike EQ and BDP, BP occurs primarily in young sexually active men in their 30s [15]. It is highly contagious, and the sexual partners of patients affected often have evidence of cervical intraepithelial neoplasia [40]. Lesions occur primarily on the penile shaft and mons pubis, although they can also occasionally arise on the glans and prepuce. They usually appear as multiple, red, velvety, maculopapular areas, which can coalesce to form larger plaques (**Figure 7.7**). The risk of malignant evolution in BP is low. But it is also known that long-standing BP can transform into BDP [41–43]. The occurrence of BP together with, or developing into, anogenital SCC has also been reported [41–45].

Giant condyloma accuminatum

Condyloma acuminata are common benign lesions. The lesions are papillomatous, papular, filiform or verrucous, exophytic growth which can affect any part of the anogenital region. On the penis, lesions typically occur around the coronal sulcus and frenulum, but can also be found as flat lesions on the penile shaft. They can occasionally extend into the

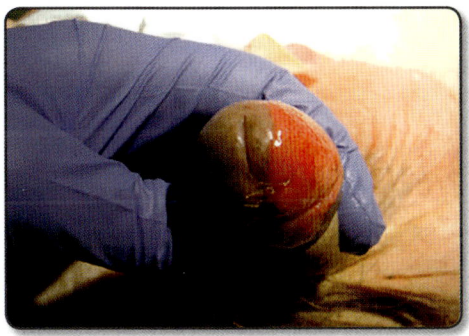

Figure 7.6 Erythroplasia of Queyrat presenting in an uncircumcised male who noticed a progressive red area on the glans penis.

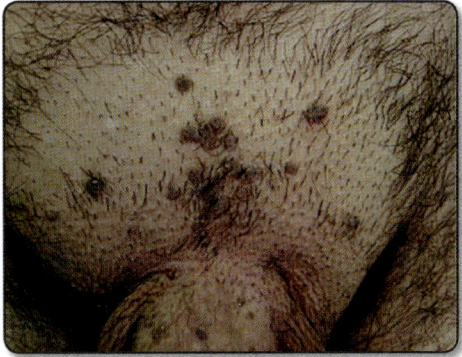

Figure 7.7 Bowenoid papulosis. Multifocal lesions are seen on the infrapubic area and penile shaft.

anterior urethra, but extension into the posterior urethra and bladder is usually only seen in immunocompromised patients [46]. They are due to infection with low-risk HPV types 6 and 11 [47–48]. These lesions typically occur in sexually active men in their third decade. Smaller lesions can be treated with topical podophyllin or trichloroacetic acid. Alternative topical treatment options include imiquimod cream. Laser therapy and cryotherapy can also be used for lesions on the glans.

Confluence of lesions can lead to the development of large, exophytic, cauliflower- like growths known as GCA (**Figure 7.8**). Risk factors for the development of GCA include immunosuppression, chronic irritation, and poor hygiene [49], and consequently they are more common in uncircumcised men. GCA is at risk of malignant transformation into invasive SCC, with reported rates between 30% and 56% [49–51]. GCA is known for its propensity for local recurrences and hence long-term follow-up is recommended.

Treatment of premalignant penile lesions

Early biopsy is important to establish the diagnosis. Premalignant disease limited to the foreskin can be treated by circumcision. Circumcision removes a major risk factor for cancer and provides more extensive tissue for histology. Often any residual disease on the glans penis tends to regress following the circumcision as there is a period of eukeratinisation of the glans penis. Topical 5-fluorouracil (5-FU) is a well-established option for the treatment of BDP, BP and EQ and can be used for small volume disease or to treat residual disease following circumcision [1,34]. Other treatments include cryosurgery, curettage and electrocautery, excisional surgery, glans resurfacing, Mohs micrographic surgery, laser and photodynamic therapy [1,34,52]. Radiotherapy should be avoided. Topical imiquimod may also be helpful [54–58]. Surgical intervention is offered for widespread PeIN by performing a glans resurfacing procedure with a split skin graft. This involves excision of the entire glans epithelium down to the level of the corpus spongiosum. Additional deep biopsies are performed to exclude invasive SCC in the corpus spongiosum.

Penile cancer

Penile cancer is a rare malignancy with just over 500 new cases in the UK per annum which accounts for less than 1% of male cancers. In the UK, the management of these tumours is now centred in specialist penile cancer units which allows patients to undergo penile preserving surgical procedures, penile reconstruction and if deemed appropriate, dynamic sentinel lymph node biopsies.

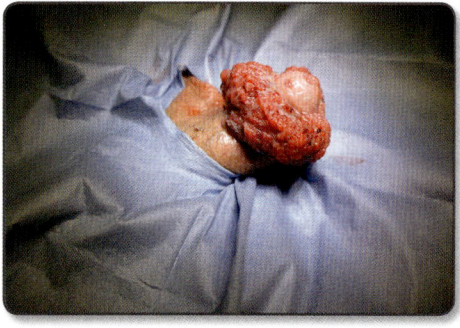

Figure 7.8 Giant condylomata acuminata in a 51-year-old patient from Eastern Europe. Presentation only occurred following voiding difficulties. Despite the extensive lesion which destroyed the glans penis and distal urethra, the corpus cavernosum was spared.

The majority of tumours are located on the glans penis (80%) or the foreskin (15%). SCC account for 95% of the tumours with the remaining 5% comprised of melanomas, sarcomas, and basal cell carcinomas.

Penile SCC can appear as a nodular, ulcerative, or an erythematous lesion, with advanced cases being clinically obvious. However, there is often a pathological phimosis covering the lesion which itself can only be palpated as a hard mass under the nonretractile foreskin. The diagnosis is confirmed by a penile biopsy and where possible, additional imaging of the penis using MRI helps to define the extent of invasion of the tumour into the distal corpus cavernosum. Patients should also have their inguinal node status evaluated both clinically and using radiological imaging, using both ultrasound and CT. When there are palpable inguinal nodes, the risk of these harbouring metastatic disease is high and either an ultrasound guided fine-needle aspiration cytology can be performed or an excisional biopsy of a palpable lymph node can be performed. Confirmation of metastatic disease within the inguinal lymph nodes will mean that the patient requires a radical inguinal lymphadenectomy. In situations where there are clinically impalpable inguinal nodes at presentation, the risk of micrometastatic disease in the inguinal nodes is approximately 20% and therefore a risk adapted approach is used to manage these patients in order to avoid overtreatment [59].

Surgical management of the primary penile tumour

A prompt diagnosis and urgent referral to a specialist penile cancer centre is required for suspicious lesions particularly if the inguinal nodes are palpable. The treatment is surgical resection although radical surgery in the form of a total penectomy or partial penectomy is rarely performed.

Current surgical practice utilises penile preserving techniques for distal penile tumours located on the glans penis which allows oncological control coupled with a reduction in the anatomical and functional morbidity.

The treatment options available depend on the site and extent of disease and can involve a circumcision for preputial tumours or a glansectomy with split skin graft reconstruction for more extensive tumours into the corpus spongiosum. Tumour extension into the distal corpus cavernosum requires a partial penectomy.

Clinicians should ensure that the glans and prepuce are fully examined in patients presenting with lesions on these areas or if they present with a palpable mass under the foreskin or bleeding or discharge. If the glans penis cannot be fully visualised due to a phimosis, the patient should be referred for an urgent circumcision and biopsy of any abnormal area. When undertaking a penile biopsy, it is essential that the sample includes the underlying corpus spongiosum to ensure that invasive SCC is detected particularly in the presence of widespread PeIN.

Key points for clinical practice

- Benign genital lesions can be normal variants.
- Suspected premalignant or malignant lesions require urgent referral to penile cancer centres for biopsy and further management.
- Circumcision is an option in refractory inflammatory conditions.
- Penile cancer can be treated by penile preserving surgical techniques.
- Impalpable inguinal lymph nodes still have a risk of harbouring micrometastatic disease and require sentinel lymph node biopsy.

REFERENCES

1. Bunker CB, Porter W. The genital, perianal and umbilical regions. In: Rook's Textbook of Dermatology, Griffiths C, Barker J, Bleiker T, Chalmers R, Creamer D, (Eds), 9th edn. Wiley-Blackwell, New York 2016.
2. Porter WM, Bunker CB. The dysfunctional foreskin. Int J STD AIDS 2001; 12:216–220.
3. Rashid RS, Shim TN. Contact dermatitis. Br Med J 2016; 30:353.
4. Edwards SK, Bunker CB, Ziller F, van der Meijden. 2013 European guideline for the management of balanoposthitis. Int J STD AIDS 2014; 25:615–626.
5. Kim GK. Seborrheic Dermatitis and *Malassezia* species. J Clin Aesthet Dermatol 2009; 2:14–17.
6. Cedeno-Laurent F, Gómez-Flores M, Mendez N, et al. New insights into HIV-1 primary skin disorders. J Int AIDS Soc 2011; 14:5.
7. Kastarinen H, Oksanen T, Okokon EO, et al. Topical anti-inflammatory agents for seborrhoeic dermatitis of the face or scalp. Cochrane Database Syst Rev 2014; 5:CD009446.
8. Parisi R, Symmons DP, Griffiths CE, Ashcroft DM. Identification and Management of Psoriasis and Associated Comorbidity (IMPACT) project team. Global epidemiology of psoriasis: a systematic review of incidence and prevalence. J Invest Dermatol 2013; 133:277–285.
9. Kim J, Krueger JG. The immunopathogenesis of psoriasis. Dermatol Clin 2015; 33:13–23.
10. Meeuwis KA, de Hullu JA, Massuger LF, et al. Genital psoriasis: A systematic literature review of this hidden skin disease. Acta Derm Venereol 2011; 91:5–11.
11. National Clinical Guideline Centre (UK). Psoriasis: assessment and management of psoriasis. London: Royal College of Physicians (UK) 2012.
12. Edmonds EV, Hunt S, Hawkins D, et al. Clinical parameters in male genital lichen sclerosus: a case series of 329 patients. J Eur Acad Dermatol Venereol 2012; 26:730–737.
13. Nelson DM, Peterson AC. Lichen sclerosus: epidemiological distribution in an equal access health care system. J Urol 2011; 185:522–525.
14. Barbagli G, Palminteri E, Baiò S, et al. Lichen sclerosus of the male genitalia and urethral stricture diseases. Urol Int 2004; 73:1–5.
15. Singh JP, Priyadarshi V, Goel HK, et al. Penile lichen sclerosus: an urologist's nightmare! – A single centre experience. Urol Ann 2015; 7:303–308.
16. Bunker CB, Patel N, Shim TN. Urinary voiding symptomatology (micro-incontinence) in male genital lichen sclerosus. Acta Derm Venereol 2013; 93:246–248.
17. Depasquale I, Park AJ, Bracka A. The treatment of balanitis xeroticca obliterans. BJU Int 2000; 86:459–465.
18. Barbagli G, Palminteri E, Mirri F, et al. Penile carcinoma in patients with genital lichen sclerosus: multicenter survey. J Urol 2006; 175:1359–1363.
19. Micali G, Nasca MR, Innocenzi D. Lichen sclerosus of the glans is significantly associated with penile carcinoma. Sex Transm Infect 2001; 77:226.
20. Nasca MR, Innocenzi D, Micali G. Penile cancer among patients with genital lichen sclerosus. J Am Acad Dermatol 1999; 41:911–914.
21. Liatsikos EN, Perimenis P, Dandinis K, et al. Lichen sclerosus et atrophicus. Findings after complete circumcision. Scand J Urol Nephrol 1997; 31:453–456.
22. Kirtschig G, Becker K, Günthert A, et al. Evidence-based (S3) guideline on (anogenital) lichen sclerosus. J Eur Acad Dermatol Venereol 2015; 29:e1–43.
23. Neill SM, Lewis FM, Tatnall FM, Cox NH. British Association of Dermatologists' guidelines for the management of lichen sclerosus. Br J Dermatol 2010; 163:672–682.
24. Bunker CB. Comments on the BAD guidelines for the management of lichen sclerosus. Br J Dermatol 2011; 164:894–895.
25. Garaffa G, Shabbir M, Christopher N, et al. The surgical management of lichen sclerosus of the glans penis: our experience and review of the literature. J Sex Med 2011; 8:1246–1253.
26. Payette MJ, Weston G, Humphrey S, et al. Lichen planus and other lichenoid dermatoses: kids are not just little people. Clin Dermatol 2015; 33:631–643.
27. Reich HL, Nguyen JT, James WD. Annular lichen planus: A case series of 20 patients. J Am Acad Dermatol 2004; 50:595–599.
28. Lacey CJ, Woodhall SC, Wikstrom A, Ross J. 2012 European guideline for the management of anogenital warts. J Eur Acad Dermatol Venereol 2013; 27:e263–270.
29. National Clinical Guideline Centre (UK). Warts-anogenital. London: Royal College of Physicians (UK) 2012.

30. Fernando I, Pritchard J, Edwards SK, Grover D. UK national guideline for the management of genital molluscum in adults, 2014 Clinical Effectiveness Group, British Association for Sexual Health and HIV. Int J STD AIDS 2015; 26:687–695.
31. van der Wouden JC, van der Sande R, van Suijlekom-Smit LW, et al. Interventions for cutaneous molluscum contagiosum. Cochrane Database Syst Rev 2009; 7:CD004767.
32. Heideman DA, Waterboer T, Pawlita M, et al. Human papillomavirus-16 is the predominant type 33. etiologically involved in penile squamous cell carcinoma. J Clin Oncol 2007; 25:4550–4556.
34. Maden C, Sherman KJ, Beckmann AM, et al. History of circumcision, medical conditions, and sexual activity and risk of penile cancer. J Natl Cancer Inst 1993; 85:19–24.
35. Porter WM, Francis N, Hawkins D, Dinneen M, Bunker CB. Penile intraepithelial neoplasia: clinical spectrum and treatment of 35 cases. Br J Dermatol 2002; 147:1159–1165.
36. Wikström A, Hedblad MA, Syrjänen S. Penile intraepithelial neoplasia: histopathological evaluation, HPV typing, clinical presentation and treatment. J Eur Acad Dermatol Venereol 2011; 26:325–330.
37. Royal College of Pathologist. Dataset for penile and distal urethral cancer histopathology reports 2015.
38. Lucia MS, MiUer GJ. Histopathology of malignant lesions of the penis. Urol Clin North Am 1992; 19:227–246.
39. Wieland U, Jurk S, Weissenborn S, et al. Erythroplasia of Queyrat: coinfection with cutaneous carcinogenic human papillomavirus type 8 and genital papillomaviruses in a carcinoma in situ. J Invest Dermatol 2000; 115:396–401.
40. Mikhail GR. Cancers, precancers, and pseudocancers on the male genitalia: a review of clinical appearances, histopathology, and management. J Dermatol Surg Oncol 1980; 6:1027–1035.
41. Obalek S, Jablonska S, Beaudenon S, Walczak L, Orth G. Bowenoid papulosis of the male and female genitalia: risk of cervical neoplasia. J Am Acad Dermatol 1986; 14:433–444.
42. Bergeron C, Naghashfar Z, Canaan C, Shah K, Fu Y, Ferenczy A. Human papillomavirus type 16 in intraepithelial neoplasia (Bowenoid papulosis) and coexistent invasive carcinoma of the vulva. Int J Gynecol Pathol 1987; 6:1–11.
43. Della Torre G, Donghi R, Longoni A, et al. HPV-DNA in intraepithelial neoplasia and carcinoma of vulva and penis. Diagn Mol Pathol 1992; 1:25–30.
44. Kato T, Saijyo S, Hatchome N, Tagami H, Kawashima M. Detection of human papIllomavirus type 16 in bowenoid papulosis and invasive carcinoma occurring in the same patient with a history of cervical carcinoma. Arch Dermatol 1998; 124:851–852.
45. Hama N, Ohtsuka T, Yamazaki S. Elevated amount of human papillomavirus 31 DNA in squamous cell carcinoma developed from bowenoid papulosis. Dermatology 2004; 209:329–332.
46. Yoneta A, Yamashita T, Jin HY, Iwasawa A, Kondo S, Jimbow K. Development of squamous cell carcinoma by two high-risk human papillomaviruses (HPVs), a novel HPV-67 and HPV-31 from bowenoid papulosis. Br J Dermatol 2000; 143:604–608.
47. Rosemberg SK. Sexually transmitted papillomaviral infection in men: an update. Dermatol Clin 1991; 9:317–331.
48. Gissmann L, De Villiers EM, Zur Hausen H. Analysis of the human genital warts (condyloma acuminate) and other genital tumor for human papillomavirus type 6 DNA. Int J Cancer 1982; 29:143–146.
49. Wells M, Robertson S, Lewis F. Squamous carcinoma arising in giant perianal condyloma associated with human papillomavirus types 6 and 11. Histopathology 1988; 12:319–323.
50. Creasman C, Haas PA, Fox TA, Balazs M. Malignant transformation of anorectal giant condyloma acuminatum (Buschke Lowenstein tumor). Dis Colon Rectum 1989; 32:481–487.
51. Chu QD, Vereridis MP, Libbey NP, Wanebo HJ. Giant condyloma acuminatum (Buschke Lowenstein tumor) of the anorectal and perianal regions. Dis Colon Rectum 1994; 37:950–957.
52. Bertram P, Treutner KH, Rubben A, et al. Invasive squamous cell carcinoma in giant anorectal condyloma (Buschke Lowenstein tumor). Langenbecks Arch Chir 1995; 380:115–118.
53. Conejo-Mir JS, Muñoz MA, Linares M, Rodriguez L, Serrano A. Carbon dioxide laser treatment of erythroplasia of Queyrat: a revisited treatment to this condition. J Eur Acad Dermatol Venereol 2005; 19:643–644.
54. Hadway P, Corbishley CM, Watkin NA. Total glans resurfacing for premalignant lesions of the penis: initial outcome data. BJU Int 2006; 98:532–536.
55. Goorney BP, Polori R. A case of Bowenoid papulosis of the penis successfully treated with topical imiquimod cream 5%. Int J STD AIDS 2004; 15:833–835.
56. Pehoushek J, Smith KJ. Imiquimod and 5% fluorouracil therapy for anal and perianal squamous cell carcinoma in situ in an HIV-1 positive man. Arch Dermatol 2001; 137:14–16.

57. Micali G, Nasca MR, De Pasquale R. Erythroplasia of Queyrat treated with imiquimod 5% cream. J Am Acad Dermatol 2006; 55:901–903.
58. Taliaferro SJ, Cohen GF. Bowen's disease of the penis treated with topical imiquimod 5% cream. J Drugs Dermatol 2008; 7:483–485.
59. Wigbels B, Luger T, Metze D. Imiquimod: a new treatment possibility in bowenoid papulosis? Hautarzt 2001; 52:128–131.
60. Horenblas S, van Tinteren H. Squamous cell carcinoma of the penis. IV. Prognostic factors of survival: analysis of tumor, nodes and metastasis classification system. J Urol 1994; 151:1239–1243.

Chapter 8

Advances in photodermatology

Ewan Eadie, Sally H. Ibbotson

INTRODUCTION

It is a fascinating and dynamic time for photodermatologists! There have been major advances in knowledge and techniques in recent years, with the promise of more yet to come. In this age of technological advances Photodermatology is ideally placed to flourish and the emphasis must continue to be on robust high quality research to inform the introduction of innovation and change in clinical practice.

With such broad subject matter it would be impossible to cover all recent advances in Photodermatology. Instead, we have chosen to focus on key publications arising in recent years, in three broad subject areas – Photosensitivity Diseases and Photodiagnostics, Therapeutics and Public Health. Within the area of photosensitivity diseases we consider new literature relating to our understanding of the presentation and pathogenesis of specific photosensitivity diseases, the evolving area of photoactive drug safety and innovative photodiagnostic techniques. We will review methods of delivery of the light-based therapies and discuss recent advances in the ultraviolet (UV) photo(chemo)therapies and Photodynamic Therapy (PDT). Finally we will present important recent developments in public health issues, notably the diverse impact of sunlight and UV radiation on health. We have excluded laser therapy in this review, as this topic is too vast to cover here. Specialist text can be sourced by the reader if they wish to increase their knowledge further in this area.

PHOTOSENSITIVITY DISEASES AND PHOTODIAGNOSTICS

The photosensitivity diseases are a heterogeneous group of diverse conditions, ranging from polymorphic light eruption (PLE), which affects 18% of Northern Europeans, to the rare orphan disease hydroa vacciniforme and the photogenodermatosis, xeroderma pigmentosum.

In the immunological photodermatosis PLE, the nature of the antigen/photoantigen(s) involved in pathogenesis remains elusive, although the microbiome may be implicated [1]. In addition, dysregulation of T cells and reduced UV-induced immune suppression may

Ewan Eadie, MSci (Hons), PhD Consultant Clinical Scientist, NHS Tayside, Photobiology Unit, Dermatology Department, NHS Tayside, Ninewells Hospital & Medical School, Dundee, UK

Sally H. Ibbotson, BSc (Hons), MBChB (Hons), MD, FRCP Professor of Photodermatology, Photobiology Unit, Dermatology Department, University of Dundee, Ninewells Hospital & Medical School, Dundee, UK. Email: s.h.ibbotson@dundee.ac.uk (for correspondence)

be implicated in PLE susceptibility. Many patients with PLE are able to achieve significant desensitisation either by natural photoadaptation or the use of photo(chemo)therapy, possibly through the mechanisms of induction of regulatory T cells, immunosuppression and mast cell infiltration [2,3]. Indeed, the role of interventions for PLE has recently been the subject of systematic review [4].

Whilst some clinical similarities may exist between PLE and actinic prurigo, the latter is best considered as a distinct entity. Our group recently reported on the detailed clinical and photobiological characteristics of 24 patients with actinic prurigo in Scotland (**Figure 8.1**). This rare condition is not limited to presentation in childhood as it can present atypically and at any age; photosensitivity may not be suspected, with resulting delays in diagnosis and significant adverse impact on quality of life [5]. Whilst there are undoubtedly strong associations between actinic prurigo and the gene locus HLA DR4, a genetic predisposition for the photosensitivity disorder chronic actinic dermatitis (CAD) has not been established. The vast majority of patients with CAD have a preceding eczema, which may be due to atopy, contact allergy or other cause. We hypothesised that impaired barrier function may predispose to UV photosensitivity in CAD, although did not show any specific association with filaggrin status [6].

Management of severe photosensitivity is a major challenge, with many patients experiencing severe adverse impact on their quality of life. The use of the IgE monoclonal antibody, omalizumab may revolutionise the life of patients with severe idiopathic solar urticaria, although lack of response in some patients supports the belief that the condition is highly heterogeneous, with several chromophores likely to be implicated [7]. The use of alpha-melanocyte stimulating hormone (α-MSH; afamelanotide) with benefit in patients with solar urticaria has been superseded by its use in erythropoietic protoporphyria, with significant improvement in tolerance of sun exposure and quality of life [8].

Diagnosis can also be a challenge and it is essential not to miss the rare photogenodermatoses, as there may be a risk of accelerated photocarcinogenesis, neurodegeneration or developmental delay, as exemplified by the condition xeroderma pigmentosum (XP). Major advances have been made in our understanding of the

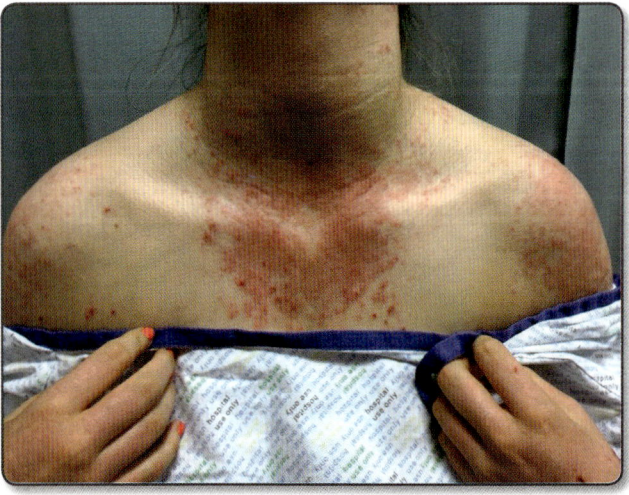

Figure 8.1 Actinic prurigo in a young female, showing the photoexposed site predominance of disease. There was delay in diagnosis as she was initially thought to have photoaggravated atopic eczema. Image by permission from (5) with adapted legend.

pathogenesis, clinical and investigative features of this rare group of diseases through the exemplary work of Fassihi and colleagues, who undertook in depth phenotyping and molecular characterisation of a unique cohort of 89 patients with XP, who had been investigated through the multidisciplinary NHS England Highly Specialist XP service. This study highlighted the importance of detection of early signs of freckling and hypopigmented macules, awareness of ocular and neurodegenerative involvement and marked heterogeneity in the disease. Invaluable predictive and prognostic information was revealed, emphasising the importance of accurate diagnosis and detailed phenotyping, strict photoprotection and vigilance (**Figure 8.2**). Interestingly, many of the patients with mild photosensitivity developed skin cancers at an earlier age than those with more severe photosensitivity, presumably due to more relaxed photoprotection [9].

Turning from rare genetic photosensitivity diseases to a much more commonplace scenario – photoactive drugs. Whilst the majority of drugs prescribed absorb ultraviolet radiation, the minority cause photosensitivity reactions [10]. Most drug-induced photosensitivity is due to phototoxicity, which may be detected through post-marketing surveillance. However, regulatory requirements for *in vitro* and *in vivo* photosafety investigations will usually highlight the potential for a drug to cause significant photosensitivity in clinical use, although this will not necessarily be a barrier to the drug's release, depending on the nature of the photosensitivity and the indication for use. The gold standard in man would be monochromator phototesting on drug, as broad band phototesting, for example with a solar simulator, may miss significant UVA and visible light photosensitivity [11].

Dermatologists may not necessarily be aware of the frequency of photosensitivity to some drugs when used in a different medical discipline. A recent example of this is the drug 5-methyl-1-phenyl-2-[1H]-pyridine, known as pirfenidone, for idiopathic pulmonary fibrosis. Despite early clinical trials indicating photosensitivity in almost half of patients taking pirfenidone, it was only with approval by the National Institute for Health and Care Excellence (NICE) in the UK in 2013, that this reached the dermatology literature [12–14]. There are other interesting observations with drug-induced photosensitivity, including voriconazole and vemurafenib [15]. Concerns have been raised about accelerated photocarcinogenesis with photoactive drugs, which was comprehensively reviewed by O'Gorman & Murphy, highlighting mechanistic insights for further study and, of course,

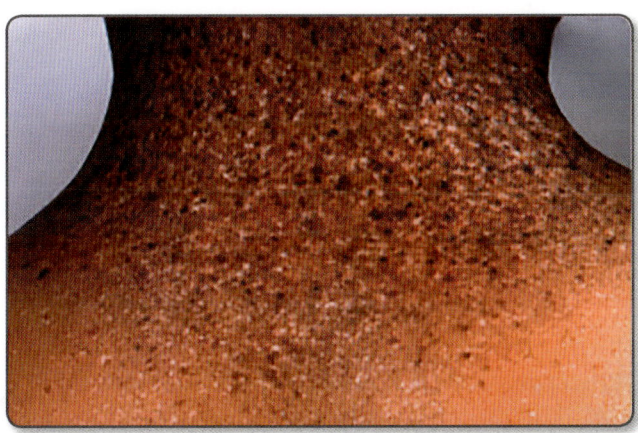

Figure 8.2 Xeroderma pigmentosum: showing the intense photo-exposed site abnormal lentigines and hypopigmented macules.

leading to possible links with chronic ingestion of photoactive drugs, such as thiazides and skin cancer and speculation with respect to possible ocular or systemic effects [16,17]. Other mechanisms for drug-induced photosensitivity may be implicated and, as a recent example, proton pump antagonist-induced lupus is increasingly recognised [18].

Investigation of patients with suspected photosensitivity may be a challenge as it requires specialist knowledge, expertise, equipment and dedicated photophysics input. The gold standard investigation is irradiation monochromator phototesting, which is only available in specialist centres. This is not ideal as it may involve patients travelling large distances. Attempts are therefore being made to introduce front line phototesting at nonspecialist centres, which has been made possible through recent advances in ultraviolet light emitting diode technology. Wan et al. have developed and validated a high intensity 365 nm LED source which is cheap, portable and could be used in rural locations or by non-specialist centres [19], with appropriate training and oversight by those with photobiology expertise.

The phototesting device mentioned above is an example of how LED technology has the potential to revolutionise the field of photodermatology. Uptake in this new technology has been slow and a commentary in 2010 predicted this, stating that a lack of commercial appetite for UV LEDs could delay the development and use of this technology in the medical sector [20]. Hopefully we will soon see similarities between the increased LED use that we have seen in the home, with that in medicine. The wide availability of LED lighting for indoor use is a welcome development for some patients with severe photosensitivity diseases. After incandescent lighting was phased out, the most available light bulb for the home was the Compact Fluorescent Lamp (CFL). However, work performed in Dundee demonstrated that the UV emissions from CFLs, coupled with the lack of heat produced thereby allowing close proximity, was of potential risk to some patients with photosensitivity diseases [21]. In the same study, no reactions were seen to the LEDs, which therefore are a safer choice for UV sensitive patients.

Photodiagnostic centres will usually also undertake detailed allergy testing, when indicated. For example, some chemicals, notably sunscreen and non-steroidal anti-inflammmatory agents, only cause allergic reactions if irradiated with UV light. Photopatch testing is thus the investigation of choice for patients with suspected photocontact allergic dermatitis to these agents, when delivered topically. European guidelines recommended a standard series of photoallergens for usage in photopatch testing, based on a large European study [22] and subsequently more recent allergens have emerged, including octocrylene, a sunscreen chemical increasingly included in sunscreen and cosmetic products and now implicated as a relatively common photoallergen, which may also be important in children [23]. Vigilance is thus required as new agents come to market.

PHOTOTHERAPEUTICS

UV-based phototherapies

Light-based therapies are essential, effective treatment options for a diverse range of skin diseases inadequately managed by topical therapies alone. Optimal use of photo(chemo) therapies, such as psoralen plus ultraviolet A radiation (PUVA), may remove the need for more toxic and often expensive drugs, including the biologics. Mechanistic studies emerging from Austria continue to delineate the pathways involved in the effects of PUVA [3]. However, in practice clinical approaches to optimised treatment regimens remain of paramount importance. Indeed, emphasis on appropriate PUVA use is recently reported in detailed PUVA guidelines undertaken in conjunction between the BAD and the BPG, which serve as an invaluable current resource for dermatologists and highlight the importance of awareness of this therapeutic approach [24]. Likewise, current guidelines relating to the use of phototherapy and PUVA for cutaneous T-cell lymphoma are also invaluable in the clinical setting [25]. Studies to identify possible individual predictive factors of response to photo(chemo)therapies have highlighted possible roles for polymorphic genes implicated in antioxidant defence, exemplified by the glutathione S-transferases, as determinants of UVB and PUVA threshold erythemal sensitivity [26]. A possible role of filaggrin as a determinant of UV sensitivity has also been investigated, given the association with impaired barrier function and immunomodulation, although interestingly, no significant association was found [27].

Optimisation of phototherapy and practicalities of treatment delivery are key objectives of treatment and will depend on the disease being treated and what is locally available. Calibration and dosimetry, with dedicated photophysics input are key aspects of successful phototherapy delivery [28]. Narrowband UVB would usually be the phototherapy of choice in most treatable diseases and ease of access and patient convenience are important as highlighted by successful delivery of both home and self-administered phototherapy [29–32]. Defining work by Weatherhead and colleagues reinforced the relative effectiveness of NBUVB for psoriasis and the important mechanisms of keratinocyte and T-cell apoptosis [33]. Whilst not available in all centres, UVA1 phototherapy is effective in specific diseases, including atopic eczema and scleroderma [34]. Historically, UVA1 has been considered to be safer than UVB or PUVA, although recent work by Tewari and colleagues has eloquently demonstrated the formation of cyclobutane pyrimidine dimers in the epidermal basal layer and dermis and induction of MMP12, raising concerns about carcinogenic and photoageing risks of UVA1 [35,36]. Importantly, action spectra studies for specific diseases are difficult to undertake and therefore data are lacking. Certainly, more information is required about optimal light-based therapeutic approaches for many diseases [37].

Towards this aim, light delivery techniques have been evolving over the years to address the shortcomings of traditional techniques. Targeted ultraviolet phototherapy is a technique for treating areas of localised disease whilst sparing normal tissue, often delivering much higher doses than would be tolerated in whole body therapy. Excimer lasers and lamps have been used for several years in this area, but newer technology is becoming available which may advance the field [38]. UV-LEDs are surely part of this progress, with preliminary data already showing their effectiveness in clearance of plaque psoriasis [39]. However, there is much further work to be done on UV-LEDs before they are powerful enough and cheap enough to be commercially viable. In the meantime, an alternative commercially available targeted digital phototherapy is available in the form of Skintrek®. Image recognition software identifies the area of affected skin to be treated prior to light being shone onto an array of tiny micro mirrors, which are angled to target only the diseased skin (**Figure 8.3**). Normal skin is completely spared and it has been shown to be as effective for psoriasis as topical PUVA and NB-UVB phototherapy [40].

Photodynamic therapy

There has been a dramatic expansion of published PDT studies recently, as the need for optimisation of treatment regimens for improved outcome and reduced adverse effects is realised [41,42]. Targeting of light delivery, to minimise pain and optimise

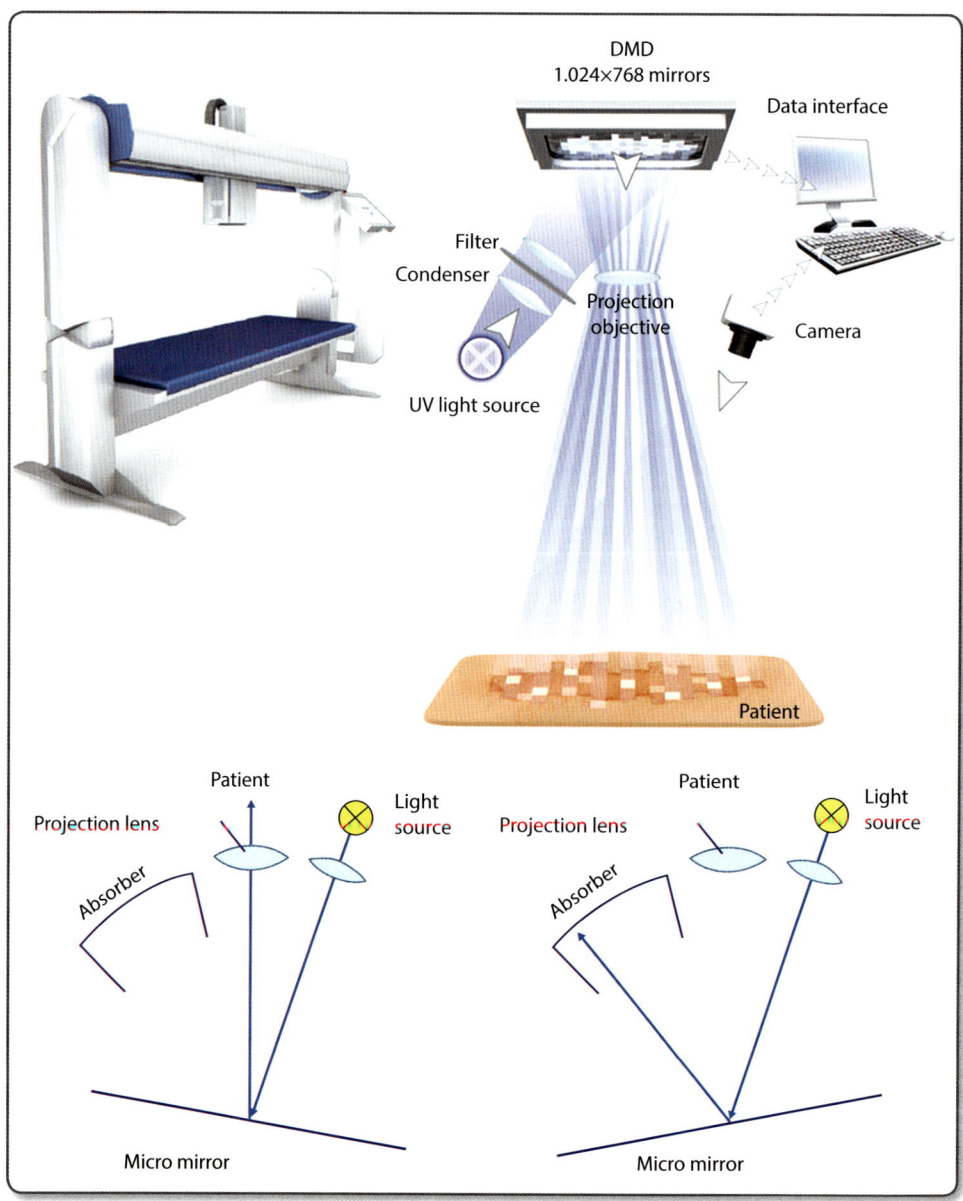

Figure 8.3 Digital phototherapy device skintrek_PT5. With permission from Friedrich Lüllau, Lüllau Engineering, Adendorf, Germany.

outcomes, is available from commercially available very low irradiance portable LED devices (**Figure 8.4**). Convenient for home use, this increases options for some patients requiring PDT. An open study of 53 patients with superficial non melanoma skin cancer and dysplasia treated with portable PDT (Ambulight, Ambicare Health Ltd.) indicated that this may be as effective, less painful and more convenient than conventional PDT [43]. Emerging data from a randomised controlled trial comparing conventional and ambulatory PDT indicate that ambulatory PDT is at least as effective and well tolerated

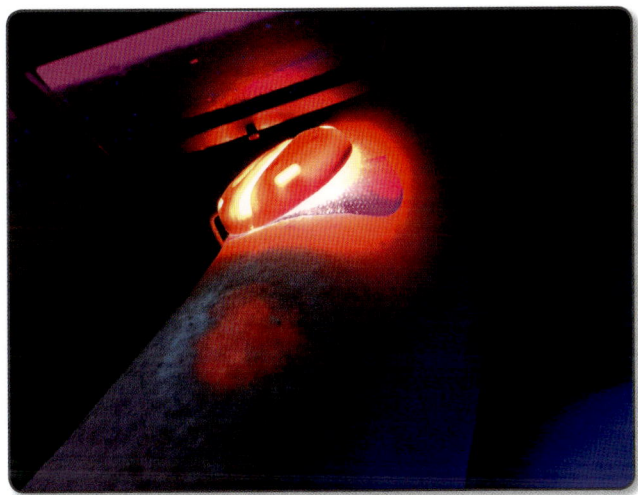

Figure 8.4 In the foreground is an image taken under Wood's light-of methylaminolevulinate-induced pprotoporphyrin IX fluorescence in photodamaged skin, whilst a separate lesion in the background is treated with PDT using the Ambulight device (Ambicare Health Ltd).

as conventional PDT for small lesions of basal cell carcinoma and Bowen's disease, with high levels of patient satisfaction. Thus, portable devices may be effectively used for PDT and are an option for improved convenience for patients [44]. Flexitheralight® is another product that delivers targeted treatment in PDT. Light is delivered through side-emitting optical fibres (SEOF) which can be woven into fabrics, worn by the patient and, in theory, will deliver a more even distribution of light compared to traditional lamps. There are no clinical data available yet for this product but the outcome of a Phase II clinical trial is imminent [45].

Much of the recent advances in light delivery as described above have focussed on portability, patient satisfaction and moving treatment out of the hospital and in to the community. Reduction in irradiance of light delivery is associated with lower pain scores during PDT. Daylight PDT is another excellent example of low irradiance, convenient, well tolerated effective treatment for field change actinic keratosis (AK), which has been shown to be as effective as but much less painful than conventional PDT for AK. First described in 2008, there is now an excellent evidence base for this treatment with European and International consensus guidelines [46–50]. A recent publication suggests that even in the variable weather conditions of the UK, daylight PDT can probably be performed at times of the year currently not considered (**Table 8.1**), particularly if a conservatory is available for use [51]. Conservatory-daylight PDT can overcome the treatment obstacle of low temperatures, although in heavy rain conditions dPDT isn't possible. Various research groups have attempted to address this issue with artificial daylight PDT – the use of indoor light sources to recreate daylight exposure conditions. Whilst these have been shown to be non-inferior, there is scope for further research in this area [52,53].

Daylight PDT has been so successful in part due to patient satisfaction with the treatment, both with convenience but importantly reduction in pain compared with conventional PDT. The treatment is feasible in the UK, even in Scotland [54]. Comparative studies indicated that daylight PDT was of similar efficacy to ingenol mebutate for mild to moderate AK, but was better tolerated [55,56]. However robust randomised comparative studies are essential in further establishing the place of PDT. One multicentre randomised comparative study of conventional PDT with imiquimod for superficial BCC indicated superior efficacy for imiquimod, although caution in interpretation is required as this was

Table 8.1 Measurement-based evidence of possible treatment times in the UK for daylight PDT. Adapted from O'Mahoney et al. [50]				
Location	**Outdoors**		**In a conservatory**	
	From	To	From	To
Lerwick	May 09:00 – 16:00	Oct 09:00 – 16:00	Feb 09:00 – 16:00	Oct 09:00 – 16:00
Inverness	Apr 09:00 – 16:00	Oct 09:00 – 16:00	Feb 09:00 – 16:00	Nov 10:00 – 15:00
Glasgow	Apr 09:00 – 16:00	Oct 09:00 – 16:00	Feb 09:00 – 16:00	Oct 09:00 – 16:00
Malin Head	Apr 09:00 – 16:00	Nov 09:00 – 16:00	Feb 09:00 – 16:00	Nov 10:00 – 15:00
Belfast	Apr 09:00 – 17:00	Nov 09:00 – 17:00	Jan 10:00 – 15:00	Nov 09:00 – 15:00
Leeds	Apr 09:00 – 16:00	Oct 09:00 – 16:00	Jan 10:00 – 15:00	Nov 09:00 – 15:00
Swansea	Apr 09:00 – 17:00	Dec 09:00 – 17:00	Jan 09:00 – 15:00	Dec 10:00 – 15:00
London	Mar 09:00 – 17:00	Dec 09:00 – 17:00	Jan 09:00 – 15:00	Dec 09:00 – 15:00
Camborne	Apr 09:00 – 17:00	Dec 09:00 – 17:00	Jan 09:00 – 16:00	Dec 10:00 – 15:00

single cycle PDT and patients unable to use imiquimod were excluded, so further studies are required [57] and both therapies may have their place for selected patients.

Daylight PDT is not a replacement for conventional PDT in certain situations and therefore alternatives for pain prevention or relief are required. Nerve blockade can be effective but is only feasible in certain sites and is relatively invasive [58]. Receptor channels TRPA1 and TRPV1 have recently been identified as being responsive to light induced oxidative stress and are implicated in PDT-induced pain mechanisms [59,60]. These receptor channels are found in pain signalling nerve endings, which opens up the possibility of targeted pain prevention and relief during PDT, but also for the cutaneous porphyrias. This requires further study and may be facilitated by non-invasive imaging of cutaneous PpIX [61].

Light delivery is one key component of PDT, with tissue-localised photosensitiser and oxygen being other critical factors for effective PDT. Recently there has been a lot of research interest in optimisation of drug delivery, with emphasis on pre-treatment regimens, such as fractional laser [62], intense pulsed lIght [63], temperature modulation [64], microneedling, topical 5-fluorouracil or salicylic acid. Choice of drug and conditions is important and randomised multicentre studies have shown increased clearance rates with the nanocolloid emulsion of ALA (BF-200, Ameluz) compared with the more widely used agent methylaminolevulinate (MAL) for mild to moderate AK [65], with maintained efficacy at 12 months (66). High clearance rates have also been reported for Ameluz PDT for field-directed treatment of mild to moderate AK, when compared with placebo [67]. However, MAL and Ameluz daylight PDT seem to be of similar efficacy and tolerability for mild to moderate AK [68], whereas hexyl-5-aminolaevulinate, although as efficacious as MAL for low grade lesions is less effective for thicker AK [69]. Interestingly, ALA impregnated in a patch may also be effective for AK and no pre-treatment is required [70], although at present patch PDT is not approved for use in the UK.

The role of topical PDT for other indications is an evolving area and one that cannot be comprehensively covered here. However, as examples, the use of PDT for selected patients with inflammatory acne vulgaris may have a place and other photosensitisers, such as indocyanine green, are under investigation [71–73]. The anti-infective effects of PDT are also of considerable interest and we suspect will be exploited further in future work [74,75].

We have some understanding of the mechanisms of effect of topical PDT in skin but biomarkers may be essential surrogates for predictors of treatment responses [76,77]. In this regard, mathematical modelling and non-invasive imaging, including in vivo fluorescence monitoring may be invaluable in facilitating optimisation of PDT regimens [78–81].

Public Health

There are undoubtedly risks and benefits associated with sun exposure and an awareness of the public health debate currently surrounding sunlight exposure levels is of fundamental importance. A balanced approach to education and advice is the subject of recent guidance from NICE [82]. Interestingly, recreational intermittent sun exposure is increasingly implicated in skin cancer risk [83,84] and therefore future developments in personal monitoring of sun exposure doses may offer patients more control of their own individual exposure risks [85]. The consequences of ozone depletion are also likely to have health implications and have recently been reviewed [86].

Sunlight, specifically UVB, provides us with our main source of Vitamin D through cutaneous photosynthesis and whilst there have been large numbers of publications on the subject, a recent overview published in the British Medical Journal stated that there was no convincing evidence of health benefits from high levels of vitamin D or from supplementation [87]. Thus, it is important to appreciate the careful balance required between cutaneous photosynthesis of vitamin D and that of the well-established skin cancer risk. Careful consideration is required with respect to advice on photoprotection and supplementation. Individual characteristics, knowledge and cultural attitudes and specific patient groups, notably those of higher skin phototype and those with photosensitivity diseases, must be taken into account as evidenced in robust clinical studies [88–92].

Of course the benefits of sun exposure are not limited to Vitamin D synthesis. Recent work has highlighted potential cardiovascular benefits of sun exposure, independent of vitamin D and further studies are required to validate these observations [93,94].

There has also been a recent increase in the interest of photoprotective properties of antioxidants and nutriceuticals , either applied topically for example with sulforaphane (broccoli) [95] or green tea extracts [96] or, as oral supplements and food sources with advantages beyond their nutritional value. Interestingly, one study of blackcurrant juice, whilst showing beneficial cardiovascular effects, did not show significant photoprotection objectively [97] and thus it is likely that combination vitamins/antioxidants and dose dependency will be relevant. A definitive study of oral nicotinamide, elegantly showed a significant reduction in the development of non-melanoma skin cancer and AK in patients taking oral nicotinamide compared with placebo. This safe, effective therapeutic approach is likely to have a major impact on patient management and ultimately we would hope in reducing skin cancer risk [98].

CONCLUSION

In the preceding text we have attempted to give the reader an overview of the key recent relevant literature in Photodermatology. The list is certainly not exhaustive, and omission from the above does not indicate work of lesser significance. Indeed what is clear from this chapter is that Photodermatology is a thriving field of active interdisciplinary research.

Publications are numerous with important discoveries being made regularly but there is more to be learned with medical, scientific and technological boundaries as yet uncrossed. The above recent advances in this field are a snapshot of where we are at this point in time and offer a glimpse of what we can expect in the future.

REFERENCES

1. Patra V, Wolf P. Microbial elements as the initial triggers in the pathogenesis of polymorphic light eruption? Exp Dermatol 2016; 25:999-1001.
2. Schweintzger N, Gruber-Wackernagel A, Reginato E, et al. Levels and function of regulatory T cells in patients with polymorphic light eruption: relation to photohardening. Br J Dermatol 2015; 173:519–526.
3. Wolf P, Byrne SN, Limon-Flores AY, Hoefler G, Ullrich SE. Serotonin signalling is crucial in the induction of PUVA-induced systemic suppression of delayed-type hypersensitivity but not local apoptosis or inflammation of the skin. Exp Dermatol 2016; 25:537–543.
4. Ling T, Cunnigham C, Rhodes S, Dawe R, Rhodes L. PD04 Cochrane systematic review: interventions in polymorphic light eruption. Br J Dermatol 2016; 175:100.
5. Macfarlane L, Hawkey S, Naasan H, Ibbotson S. Characteristics of actinic prurigo in Scotland: 24 cases seen between 2001 and 2015. Br J Dermatol 2016;174:1411–1414.
6. Harkins CP, Waters A, Kerr A, et al. Loss-of-Function Mutations in the Gene Encoding Filaggrin Are Not Strongly Associated with Chronic Actinic Dermatitis. J Invest Dermatol 2015; 135:1919–1921.
7. Aubin F, Avenel-Audran M, Jeanmougin M, et al. Omalizumab in patients with severe and refractory solar urticaria: A phase II multicentric study. J Am Acad Dermatol 2016; 74:574–575.
8. Langendonk JG, Balwani M, Anderson KE, et al. Afamelanotide for Erythropoietic Protoporphyria. N Engl J Med 2015; 373:48–59.
9. Fassihi H, Sethi M, Fawcett H, et al. Deep phenotyping of 89 xeroderma pigmentosum patients reveals unexpected heterogeneity dependent on the precise molecular defect. Proc Natl Acad Sci 2016; 113:E1236 –1245.
10. Dawe RS, Ibbotson SH. Drug-induced photosensitivity. Dermatologic Clinics 2014; 32:363–368.
11. Bauer D, Soon RL, Kulmatycki K, et al. The DGAT1 inhibitor pradigastat does not induce photosensitivity in healthy human subjects: a randomized controlled trial using three defined sunlight exposure conditions. Photochem Photobiol Sci 2016; 15:1155–1162.
12. Reinholz M, Eder I, Przybilla B, et al. Photoallergic contact dermatitis due to treatment of pulmonary fibrosis with pirfenidone. J Eur Acad Dermatol Venereol 2016; 30:370–371.
13. Caruana DM, Wylie G. Cutaneous reactions to pirfenidone: a new kid on the block. Br J Dermatol 2016; 175:425–426.
14. Papakonstantinou E, Prasse A, Schacht V, Kapp A, Raap U. Pirfenidone-induced severe phototoxic reaction in a patient with idiopathic lung fibrosis. J Eur Acad Dermatol Venereol 2016; 30:1354–1356.
15. Woods JA, Ferguson JS, Kalra S, et al. The phototoxicity of vemurafenib: An investigation of clinical monochromator phototesting and in vitro phototoxicity testing. J Photochem Photobiol B 2015; 151:233–238
16. O'Gorman SM, Murphy GM. Photoaggravated Disorders. Dermatologic Clinics 2016; 32:385–398.
17. de Vries E, Trakatelli M, Kalabalikis D, Ferrandiz L, Ruiz-de-Casas A, Moreno-Ramirez D, et al. Known and potential new risk factors for skin cancer in European populations: a multicentre case-control study. The Br J Dermatol 2012; 167:1–13
18. Hung R, Sangle SR, Benton E, D'Cruz DP, McGibbon D. Proton pump inhibitor-induced subcutaneous lupus erythematosus in a patient with systemic lupus erythematosus. Clin Exp Dermatol 2015; 40:808–809.
19. Wan P, Edwards C, Zheng J, Anstey A. Validation of a novel high-intensity LED light source for skin phototesting at 365 nm. Photodermatol Photoimmunol Photomed 2012; 28:80–83
20. Edwards C, Anstey AV. Therapeutic ultraviolet light-emitting diode sources: a new phase in the evolution of phototherapy. Br J Dermatol 2010; 163:3–4.
21. Fenton L, Ferguson J, Ibbotson S, Moseley H. Energy saving lamps and their impact on photosensitive and normal individuals. Br J Dermatol 2013; 169:910–915.
22. Kerr AC, Ferguson J, Haylett AK, Rhodes LE, Adamski H, Alomar A, et al. A European Multi-centre Photopatch Test Study (EMCPPTS). Br J Dermatol 2012; 166:1002–1009

23. Manová E, von Goetz N, Hungerbühler K. Ultraviolet filter contact and photocontact allergy: consumer exposure and risk assessment for octocrylene from personal care products and sunscreens. Br J Dermatol 2014; 171:1368–1374.

24. Ling TC, Clayton TH, Crawley J, et al. British Association of Dermatologists and British Photodermatology Group guidelines for the safe and effective use of psoralen-ultraviolet A therapy 2015. Br J Dermatol 2016; 174:24–55.

25. Olsen EA, Hodak E, Anderson T, et al. Guidelines for phototherapy of mycosis fungoides and Sezary syndrome: A consensus statement of the United States Cutaneous Lymphoma Consortium. J Am Acad Dermatol 2016; 74:27–58.

26. Ibbotson SH, Dawe RS, Dinkova-Kostova AT, et al. Glutathione S-transferase genotype is associated with sensitivity to psoralen-ultraviolet A photochemotherapy. Br J Dermatol 2012; 166:380–388.

27. Forbes D, Johnston L, Gardner J, et al. Filaggrin genotype does not determine the skin's threshold to UV-induced erythema. J Allergy Clin Immunol 2016; 137:1280–1282.e3.

28. Moseley H, Allan D, Amatiello H, et al. Guidelines on the measurement of ultraviolet radiation levels in ultraviolet phototherapy: report issued by the British Association of Dermatologists and British Photodermatology Group 2015. Br J Dermatol 2015; 173:333–350.

29. Arzpayma P, Jones H, Harper P, et al. Creation and assessment of a computerized modeling tool for optimizing planning of home and hospital-based phototherapy. Br J Dermatol 2017; 176:1390–1391.

30. Yule S, Sanyal S, Ibbotson S, Moseley H, Dawe RS. Self-administration of hospital-based narrowband uvb (tl-01) phototherapy: a feasibility study in an outpatient setting. Br J Dermatol 2013; 169:464–468.

31. Cameron H, Yule S, Dawe RS, Ibbotson SH, Moseley H, et al. Review of an established UK home phototherapy service 1998-2011: improving access to a cost-effective treatment for chronic skin disease. Public Health 2014; 128:317–324.

32. Koek MB, Buskens E, van Weelden H, et al. Home versus outpatient ultraviolet B phototherapy for mild to severe psoriasis: pragmatic multicentre randomised controlled non-inferiority trial (PLUTO study). Br Med J 2009; 338:b1542.

33. Weatherhead SC, Farr PM, Jamieson D, et al. Keratinocyte apoptosis in epidermal remodeling and clearance of psoriasis induced by UV radiation. J Invest Dermatol 2011; 131:1916–1926.

34. Kerr AC, Ferguson J, Attili SK, et al. Ultraviolet A1 phototherapy: a British Photodermatology Group workshop report. Clin Exp Dermatol 2012; 37:219–226

35. Tewari A, Sarkany RP, Young AR. UVA1 Induces Cyclobutane Pyrimidine Dimers but Not 6-4 Photoproducts in Human Skin In Vivo. J Invest Dermatol 2012; 132:394–400.

36. Tewari A, Grys K, Kollet J, Sarkany R, Young AR. Upregulation of MMP12 and its activity by UVA1 in human skin: potential implications for photoaging. J Invest Dermatol 2014; 134:2598–2609.

37. Barbaric J, Abbott R, Posadzki P, et al. Light therapies for acne. Cochrane Database Syst Rev 2016; 9:CD007917

38. Alshiyab D, Edwards C, Chin MF, Anstey AV. Targeted ultraviolet B phototherapy: definition, clinical indications and limitations. Clin Exp Dermatol 2015; 40:1–5.

39. Kemeny L, Csoma Z, Bagdi E, et al. Targeted phototherapy of plaque-type psoriasis using ultraviolet B-light-emitting diodes. Br J Dermatol 2010; 163:167–173.

40. Werfel T, Holiangu F, Niemann KH, et al. Digital ultraviolet therapy: a novel therapeutic approach for the targeted treatment of psoriasis vulgaris. Br J Dermatol 2015; 172:746–753.

41. Wiegell SR, Lerche CM, Wulf HC. Is the thin layer of methyl aminolevulinate used during photodynamic therapy sufficient? Photodermatol Photoimmunol Photomed 2016; 32:88–92

42. Wiegell SR, Petersen B, Wulf HC. Pulse photodynamic therapy reduces inflammation without compromising efficacy in the treatment of multiple mild actinic keratoses of the face and scalp: a randomized clinical trial. Br J Dermatol 2016; 174:979–984.

43. Ibbotson S, Ferguson J. Ambulatory photodynamic therapy using low irradiance inorganic light-emitting diodes for the treatment of non-melanoma skin cancer: an open study. Photodermatol Photoimmunol Photomed 2012; 28:235–239.

44. Ibbotson SH, Dawe RS, Moseley H, Samuel IDW, Ferguson J. A randomised, controlled trial of portable compared with conventional photodynamic therapy for superficial non-melanoma skin cancer. Br J Dermatol 2018.

45. Mordon S, Cochrane C, Tylcz JB, et al. Light emitting fabric technologies for photodynamic therapy. Photodiagnosis Photodyn Ther 2015; 12:1–8.

46. Morton CA, Wulf HC, Szeimies RM, et al. Practical approach to the use of daylight photodynamic therapy with topical methyl aminolevulinate for actinic keratosis: a European consensus. . J Europ Acad Dermatol Venereol 2015; 29:1718–1723.

47. Wiegell SR, Wulf HC, Szeimies RM, et al. Daylight photodynamic therapy for actinic keratosis: an international consensus. . J Eur Acad Dermatol Venereol 2012; 26:673–679.
48. Philipp-Dormston WG, Sanclemente G, et al. Daylight photodynamic therapy with MAL cream for large-scale photodamaged skin based on the concept of `actinic field damage': recommendations of an international expert group. J Eur Acad Dermatol Venereol 2016; 30:8–15
49. Rubel DM, Spelman L, Murrell DF, et al. Daylight photodynamic therapy with methyl aminolevulinate cream as a convenient, similarly effective, nearly painless alternative to conventional photodynamic therapy in actinic keratosis treatment: a randomized controlled trial. Br J Dermatol 2014; 171:1164–1171
50. Lacour JP, Ulrich C, Gilaberte Y, et al. Daylight photodynamic therapy with methyl aminolevulinate cream is effective and nearly painless in treating actinic keratoses: a randomised, investigator-blinded, controlled, phase III study throughout Europe. J Europ Acad Dermatol Venereol 2015; 29:2342–2348.
51. O'Mahoney P, Khazova M, Higlett M, et al. The use of illuminance as a guide to effective light delivery during daylight PDT in the UK. Br J Dermatol 2017; 176:1607–1616.
52. O'Gorman SM, Clowry J, Manley M, et al. Artificial white light vs daylight photodynamic therapy for actinic keratoses: A randomized clinical trial. J Am Acad Dermatol 2016; 152:638–644
53. Lerche CM, Heerfordt IM, Heydenreich J, Wulf HC. Alternatives to Outdoor Daylight Illumination for Photodynamic Therapy -Use of Greenhouses and Artificial Light Sources. Int J Mol Sci 2016; 17:309.
54. Cordey H, Valentine R, Lesar A, et al. Daylight Photodynamic Therapy in Scotland. Scottish Med J 2017; 62:48–53
55. Moggio E, Arisi M, Calzavara-Pinton P. A randomized split-face clinical trial of daylight photodynamic therapy with methyl aminolaevulinate vs ingenol mebutate gel for the treatment of multiple actinic keratoses of the face and scalp. Photodiagnosis Photodyn Ther 2016; 16:161–165.
56. Genovese G, Fai D, Fai C, Mavilia L, Mercuri SR. Daylight methyl-aminolevulinate photodynamic therapy versus ingenol mebutate for the treatment of actinic keratoses: an intraindividual comparative analysis. Dermatol Ther 2016; 29:191–196
57. Roozeboom MH, Arits AH, Mosterd K, et al. Three-Year Follow-Up Results of Photodynamic Therapy vs. Imiquimod vs. Fluorouracil for Treatment of Superficial Basal Cell Carcinoma: A Single-Blind, Noninferiority, Randomized Controlled Trial. J Invest Dermatol 2016; 136:1568–1574
58. Klein A, Karrer S, Horner C, et al. Comparing cold-air analgesia, systemically administered analgesia and scalp nerve blocks for pain management during photodynamic therapy for actinic keratosis of the scalp presenting as field concretization: a randomized controlled trial. Br J Dermatol 2015; 173:192 -200.
59. Babes A, Sauer SK, Moparthi L, et al. Photosensitization in Porphyria's and Photodynamic Therapy Involves TRPA1 and TRPV1. J Neurosci 2016; 36:5264–5278.
60. Wright L, Baptista-Hon D, Bull F, et al. Menthol reduces phototoxicity pain in a mouse model of photodynamic therapy. Pain 2018;159:284–297.
61. Heerfordt IM, Wulf HC. Protoporphyrin IX in the skin measured non-invasively predicts photosensitivity in patients with erythropoietic protoporphyria. Br J Dermatol 2016; 175:1284–1289.
62. Haak CS, Togsverd-Bo K, Thaysen-Petersen D, et al. Fractional laser-mediated photodynamic therapy of high-risk basal cell carcinomas - a randomized clinical trial. Br J Dermatol 2015; 172:215–222.
63. Kohl E, Popp C, Zeman F, et al. Photodynamic therapy using intense pulsed light for treating actinic keratoses and photoaged skin of the dorsal hands: a randomized placebo-controlled study. Br J Dermatol 2017; 176:852–362.
64. Willey A, Anderson RR, Sakamoto FH. Temperature-Modulated Photodynamic Therapy for the Treatment of Actinic Keratosis on the Extremities: A One-Year Follow-up Study. Dermatol Surg 2015; 41:1290–1295.
65. Dirschka T, Radny P, Dominicus R, et al. Photodynamic therapy with BF-200 ALA for the treatment of actinic keratosis: results of a multicentre, randomized, observer-blind phase III study in comparison to a registered methyl-5-aminolaevulinate cream and placebo. Br J Dermatol 2012; 166:137–146.
66. Dirschka T, Radny P, Dominicus R, et al. Long-term (6 and 12 months) follow-up of two prospective, randomized, controlled phase III trials of photodynamic therapy with BF-200 ALA and methyl aminolaevulinate for the treatment of actinic keratosis. Br J Dermatol 2013; 168:825–836.
67. Reinhold U, Dirschka T, Ostendorf R, et al. A randomized, double-blind, phase III, multicentre study to evaluate the safety and efficacy of BF-200 ALA (Ameluz®) vs. placebo in the field-directed treatment of mild-to-moderate actinic keratosis with photodynamic therapy (PDT) when using the BF-RhodoLED® lamp. Br J Dermatol 2016; 175:696–705.
68. Neittaanmäki-Perttu N, Karppinen TT, Grönroos M, Tani TT, Snellman E. Daylight photodynamic therapy for actinic keratoses: a randomized double-blinded nonsponsored prospective study comparing 5-aminolaevulinic acid nanoemulsion (BF-200) with methyl-5-aminolaevulinate. Br J Dermatol 2014; 171:1172–1180.

69. Neittaanmäki-Perttu N, Grönroos M, Karppinen TT, Tani TT, Snellman E. Hexyl-5-aminolaevulinate 0·2% vs. methyl-5-aminolaevulinate 16% daylight photodynamic therapy for treatment of actinic keratoses: results of a randomized double-blinded pilot trial. Br J Dermatol 2016; 174:427–429.

70. Szeimies RM, Hauschild A, Ortland C, Moor ACE, Stocker M, Surber C. Photodynamic therapy simplified: nonprepared, moderate-grade actinic keratosis lesions respond equally well to 5-aminolaevulinic acid patch photodynamic therapy as do mild lesions. Br J Dermatol 2015; 173:1277–1279.

71. Keyal U, Bhatta AK, Wang XL. Photodynamic therapy for the treatment of different severity of acne: A systematic review. Photodiagnosis Photodyna Ther 2016; 14:191–199.

72. Taylor M. Photodynamic therapy for acne: are we there yet? Br J Dermatol 2016; 174:712–713.

73. Seo H, Min H, Kim H, et al. Effects of repetitive photodynamic therapy using indocyanine green for acne vulgaris. Int J Dermatol 2016; 55:1157–1163.

74. Bhatta AK, Keyal U, Wang XL. Photodynamic therapy for onychomycosis: A systematic review. Photodiagnosis Photodyn Ther 2016; 15:228–235.

75. Gilaberte Y, Robres MP, Frías MP, et al. Methyl aminolevulinate photodynamic therapy for onychomycosis: a multicentre, randomized, controlled clinical trial. J Eur Acad Dermatol Venereol 2017; 31:347–354.

76. Mills SJ, Farrar MD, Ashcroft GS, et al. Topical photodynamic therapy following excisional wounding of human skin increases production of transforming growth factor-beta3 and matrix metalloproteinases 1 and 9, with associated improvement in dermal matrix organization. Br J Dermatol 2014; 171:55–62.

77. Brooke RC, Sidhu M, Sinha A, et al. Prostaglandin E2 and nitric oxide mediate the acute inflammatory (erythemal) response to topical 5-aminolaevulinic acid photodynamic therapy in human skin. Br J Dermatol 2013; 169:645–652.

78. Kulyk O, Ibbotson SH, Moseley H, Valentine RM, Samuel IDW. Development of a handheld fluorescence imaging device to investigate the characteristics of protoporphyrin IX fluorescence in healthy and diseased skin. Photodiagnosis Photodyn Ther 2015; 12:630–639.

79. Campbell CL, Brown CT, Wood K, Moseley H. Modelling topical photodynamic therapy treatment including the continuous production of Protoporphyrin IX. Phys Med Biol 2016; 61:7507–7521.

80. Campbell CL, Wood K, Brown CT, Moseley H. Monte Carlo modelling of photodynamic therapy treatments comparing clustered three dimensional tumour structures with homogeneous tissue structures. Phys Med Biol 2016; 61:4840–4854.

81. Seyed Jafari SM, Timchik T, Hunger RE. In vivo confocal microscopy efficacy assessment of daylight photodynamic therapy in actinic keratosis patients. Br J Dermatol 2016; 175:375–381.

82. National Institute for Health and Care Excellence (NICE). Sunlight exposure: risks and benefits. NICE Guideline 2016 9; 34:1–39.

83. Petersen B, Wulf HC, Triguero-Mas M, et al. Sun and ski holidays improve vitamin D status, but are associated with high levels of DNA damage. J Invest Dermatol 2014; 134:2806–2813.

84. Bodekaer M, Philipsen PA, Petersen B, Heydenreich J, Wulf HC. Defining "intermittent UVR exposure". Photochem Photobiol Sci 2016; 15:1176–1182.

85. Morelli M, Masini A, Simeone E, Khazova M. Validation and in vivo assessment of an innovative satellite-based solar UV dosimeter for a mobile app dedicated to skin health. Photochem Photobiolog Sci 2016; 15:1170–1175.

86. Lucas RM, Norval M, Neale RE, et al. The consequences for human health of stratospheric ozone depletion in association with other environmental factors. Photochem Photobiolog Sci 2015; 14:53–87.

87. Theodoratou E, Tzoulaki I, Zgaga L, Ioannidis JP. Vitamin D and multiple health outcomes: umbrella review of systematic reviews and meta-analyses of observational studies and randomised trials. Br Med J 2014; 348:g2035.

88. Rhodes LE, Webb AR, Berry JL, et al. Sunlight exposure behaviour and vitamin D status in photosensitive patients: longitudinal comparative study with healthy individuals at UK latitude. Br J Dermatol 2014; 171:1478–1486.

89. Felton SJ, Cooke MS, Kift R, et al. Concurrent beneficial (vitamin D production) and hazardous (cutaneous DNA damage) impact of repeated low-level summer sunlight exposures. Br J Dermatol 2016; 175:1320–1328.

90. Webb AR, Aseem S, Kift RC, Rhodes LE, Farrar MD. Target the message: A qualitative study exploring knowledge and cultural attitudes to sunlight and vitamin D in Greater Manchester, UK. Br J Dermatol 2016; 175:4101–1403.

91. Fajuyigbe D, Young AR. The impact of skin colour on human photobiological responses. Pigment Cell & Melanoma Res 2016; 29:607–618.

92. Datta P, Philipsen PA, Olsen P, Petersen B, Johansen P, Morling N, et al. Major inter-personal variation in the increase and maximal level of 25-hydroxy vitamin D induced by UVB. Photochem Photobiolog Sci 2016; 15:536–545.

93. Weller RB. Sunlight Has Cardiovascular Benefits Independently of Vitamin D. Blood Purif 2016; 41:130–134.
94. Liu D, Fernandez BO, Hamilton A, et al. UVA irradiation of human skin vasodilates arterial vasculature and lowers blood pressure independently of nitric oxide synthase. J Invest Dermatol 2014; 134:1839–1846.
95. Knatko EV, Ibbotson SH, Zhang Y, et al. Nrf2 Activation Protects against Solar-Simulated Ultraviolet Radiation in Mice and Humans. Cancer Prev Res (Phila) 2015; 8:475–486.
96. Farrar MD, Nicolaou A, Clarke KA, et al. A randomized controlled trial of green tea catechins in protection against ultraviolet radiation-induced cutaneous inflammation. Am J Clin Nutr 2015; 102:608–615.
97. Ray S, Belch JJ, Craigie AM, et al. Can antioxidant-rich blackcurrant juice drink consumption improve photoprotection against ultraviolet radiation? Br J Dermatol 2016; 174:1101–1103.
98. Chen AC, Martin AJ, Choy B, et al. A Phase 3 Randomized Trial of Nicotinamide for Skin-Cancer Chemoprevention. N Engl J Med 2015; 373:1618–1626.

Chapter 9

Advances in Mohs surgery

Miriam Fitzgerald, James Shelley

INTRODUCTION

Mohs micrographic surgery (MMS) is a highly specialised type of surgery used to treat an array of complex skin cancers. It offers the distinct advantages of complete microscopic margin control coupled with tissue conservation and leads to high cure rates [1].

It was first developed by Dr Frederic Edward Mohs in 1936 while he was a medical student at the University of Wisconsin. MMS is currently the most precise tissue-sparing method for the treatment of basal cell carcinomas (BCC) and squamous cell carcinomas (SCC) which are the most common cancers worldwide [2].

HISTORY/BACKGROUND

Frederic Edward Mohs (1910–2002) was a medical student at the University of Wisconsin, Madison from 1929–1934. In 1933, 23-year-old Frederic was a research assistant assigned to inject different chemicals into cancerous rat tissues to produce specific reactions. He discovered that one of these chemicals, a zinc chloride solution, could 'fix' skin tissue for microscopic study — preserve it without changing the architectural structure of the cells [3].

Creating a zinc chloride-containing paste, Mohs discovered that tissue could be excised precisely with minimal bleeding. These specimens were subsequently prepared as frozen sections ready for viewing under the microscope. After training as a surgeon, Mohs began using the technique of 'chemosurgery' (so-called due to the zinc chloride paste) on human skin cancer patients in 1936. The initial process took several days. It involved clinically identifying a skin cancer, applying dichloroacetic acid to the involved area and curettage of the epidermal keratin layer to allow the zinc chloride paste to penetrate. To enhance tissue absorption of the paste a protective dressing was then applied. Drawbacks included the painful and time-consuming nature of the process and devitalisation of wound edges due to the zinc chloride paste [4] which therefore negated the possibility of immediate reconstruction.

Miriam Fitzgerald MBBCh BAO(Hons) MRCP(UK) MRCP(Ireland) Dermatology Registrar, Chelsea and Westminster Hospital, London, UK

James Shelley MB BS FRCP MRCSEd, Consultant dermatologist and Mohs surgeon, Chelsea and Westminster Hospital, London, UK. Email: James.Shelley@chelwest.nhs.uk (for correspondence)

Mohs' landmark article on 440 patients treated with chemosurgery appeared in the Archives of Surgery in 1941 [5]. Problems encountered after testing the chemosurgical technique included ocular damage when treating eyelid tumours. In 1953, Mohs discovered a solution to this problem and subsequently developed the 'fresh-tissue technique'. This involved infiltrating the area with local anaesthetic and excising the affected tissue straight after, in a horizontal or tangential manner, the frozen sections of which were then analysed under the microscope. This minimised pain caused by tissue fixation on the skin, multiple stages could be performed in one day and the defects could be closed immediately once tumour-free margins were achieved. The fresh-tissue technique dramatically reduced the procedure time.

INDICATIONS FOR MOHS SURGERY

Mohs micrographic surgery is primarily used to treat BCC and SCC but can be used to resect other rarer forms of skin cancer (see **Table 9.1**).

Candidates for surgery include those with recurrent BCC or high-risk primary tumours with one or more of the following features; aggressive histologic growth pattern (e.g. morphoeic BCC, anaplastic SCC), cutaneous neoplasms with poorly defined margins, location at anatomic sites for which the risk of recurrence with conventional treatment modalities is higher, location at sites requiring tissue conservation for optimal reconstruction (e.g. eyelids, nose, ears and lips), tumours > 2 cm, recurrent or incompletely excised tumours and those that display rapid growth. MMS should also be considered in patients who are immunosuppressed and in young patients (e.g. with certain genodermatosis that may predispose the development of further skin cancers in the future).

Certain other tumours can also be excised by this technique including extramammary Paget's disease, dermatofibrosarcoma protuberans, sebaceous carcinoma, atypical fibroxanthoma and malignant melanoma.

Table 9.1 Indications for Mohs micrographic surgery	
Indications for Mohs micrographic surgery	
Aggressive histological subtypes/features	Morphoeic
	Infiltrating Micronodular Basosquamous
	Perineural invasion Poorly differentiated
Sites	Nose Paranasal folds Periocular Ears Lips Scalp Genitals
Other factors	Size >2 cm Recurrent tumour Ill-defined margins Genetic disorder (e.g. Gorlin's syndrome) Immunosuppression Radiated skin

While numerous other treatment modalities are in existence for nonmelanomatous skin cancers (NMSC) including traditional surgical excision, radiation therapy, curettage and cautery, cryosurgery, photodynamic therapy and topical chemotherapeutic agents, MMS has many advantages (see advantages section below).

Although MMS is the gold standard for the treatment of NMSC, the method should be used wisely and according to the proper indications [6].

PREOPERATIVE CONSIDERATIONS

As for any surgical procedure, documenting each patient's medical and surgical history as well as medicaments and allergies is vital. In particular, attention should be paid to confirming a history of diabetes mellitus, cardiovascular or pulmonary compromise, the presence of a pacemaker or implantable cardioverter-defibrillator (ICD), history of keloid scarring, thrombocytopaenic and haemophilic states. The temporary withholding or dose reduction of medications such as aspirin, warfarin, antiplatelet medications, novel anticoagulants (such as rivaroxaban and apixaban), nonsteroidal anti-inflammatory drugs and immunosuppressants should be considered by the treating clinician at the initial Mohs assessment clinic appointment. A preoperative swab for methicillin-resistant *Staphylococcus aureus* (MRSA) may also be indicated depending on local hospital policies. Prophylactic antibiotics are not usually advocated by Mohs surgeons however this also depends on local policy, wound site and patient factors.

Consulting with other colleagues should be anticipated during the initial clinic assessment. The size, location and histologic subtype of the tumour will dictate if multidisciplinary input is required. Input from oculoplastic, plastic, haematology and dermatopathology teams are frequently required. This should be arranged and coordinated by the Mohs team well in advance of surgery.

It is often useful to provide a patient information leaflet regarding Mohs surgery to patients at their initial assessment.

THE PROCEDURE

Step 1 – The tumour is outlined and marked. Local anaesthetic is subsequently administered.

Step 2 – A curette or scalpel is used to delineate and 'debulk' the tumour.

Step 3 – The tumour is excised along with a small margin of normal tissue. This is done circumferentially with the scalpel angled at 45° to the skin (this bevels the edge to facilitate histologic processing) then parallel to the skin for the deep margin so that this part is excised horizontally.

Step 4 – Mapping of the tumour occurs, usually with colour-coded ink, to allow precise orientation of the specimen to local landmarks (e.g. nose, cheek).

Step 5 – Haemostasis is achieved (e.g. manual pressure, electrocautery).

Step 6 – A two-dimensional map is drawn of defect including corresponding orientation markers.

Step 7 – The tissue is then divided along the markings and inverted so that the dermis is now facing up. Tissue dyes are used to colour code the specimen edges.

Step 8 – The specimen is mounted with care taken to flatten the under surface before freezing in a cryostat and cutting into 5–7 nanometer horizontal sections which are placed onto slides (see **Figure 9.1**).

Step 9 – The slides are subsequently stained (most commonly with haematoxylin–eosin and toluidine blue) and viewed under the microscope by the Mohs surgeon.

Step 10 – Residual tumour is removed by repeating the process above before reconstruction of the defect, once all neoplastic cells have been resected (see **Figure 9.2**).

WOUND CLOSURE AND POSTOPERATIVE CARE

There are a number of options for closure of the defect once all of the tumour has been resected. Fellowship-trained Mohs surgeons are experts in undertaking defect reconstructions. The closure method chosen depends on the patient, the wound and its location and may not be confirmed until the residual tumour has been removed (the final defect may not be predicted prior to surgery). Healing by secondary intention, whereby the wound is left to heal naturally is often chosen. This is done in conjunction with strict wound care measures which are particularly important for the initial stages of healing. Other options include side-to-side closure, the use of flaps or skin grafts. Side-to-side closures are commonly used for smaller wounds. Flaps involve the use of skin adjacent to the surgical site to close the defect as opposed to grafts which are taken from a separate 'noncosmetic' site requiring closure of a second wound at the donor site.

Apart from inevitable scarring, which is often well disguised along the natural skin creases, patients should be counselled to expect bruising, swelling and tightening

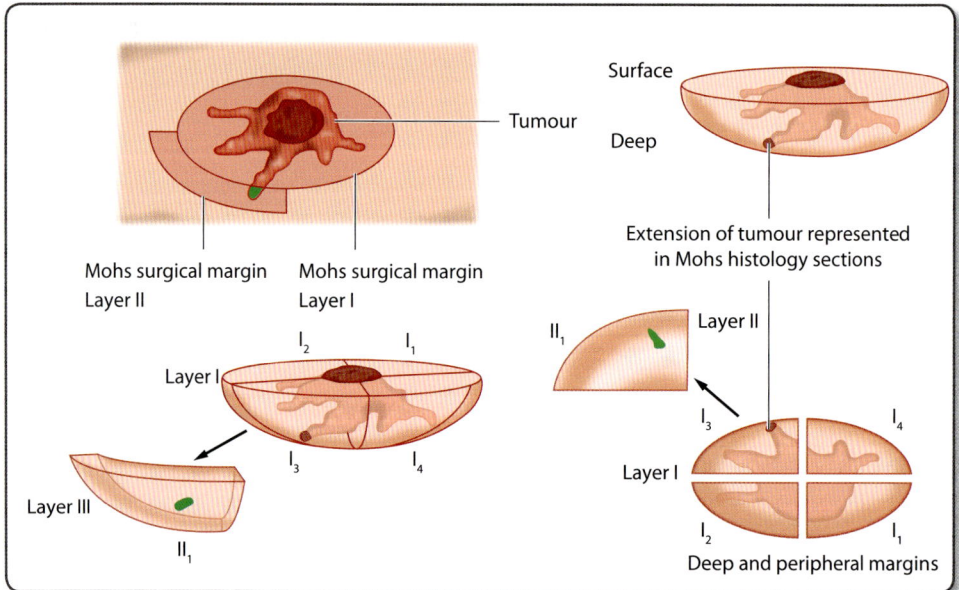

Figure 9.1 Residual tumour is removed in subsequent layers after initial debulking. Prior tumour marking (see Step 4) is essential for successful completion of this process.

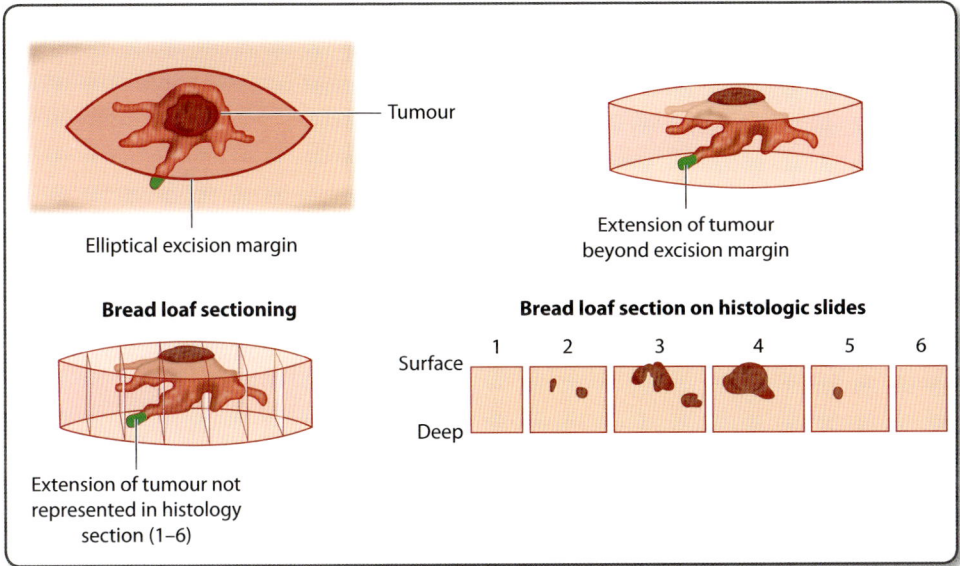

Figure 9.2 Standard processing (so-called 'bread loaf' slicing) only examines a limited portion of the tumour margins as opposed to Mohs surgery which examines one hundred percent of the margins (using horizontal sectioning).

at the surgical site all of which are usually temporary. Other potential postoperative complications include bleeding, infection, nerve damage and wound dehiscence.

THE TEAM

Mohs surgeons are most often consultant dermatologists who have completed additional fellowship training in advanced skin surgery and Mohs surgery. These surgeons are highly trained and skilled consultants who should be competent in multiple techniques including surgical excision of the tumour, pathologic examination of the specimen and advanced reconstruction techniques of the skin. National organisations such as the British Society for Dermatological Surgery (BSDS) in the United Kingdom and the American College of Mohs Surgery (ACMS) in America govern this practice.

As per BSDS guideline recommendations [7] the MMS team should also consist of a surgical assistant who also provides pre- and postoperative as well as wound care advice. Skilled laboratory technicians are imperative for the successful processing of slides which includes tissue fixation, freezing, precise cutting of nanometer sections in the cryostat and tissue staining. A dermatopathologist is another member of the multidisciplinary team who may subsequently report on the Mohs surgeon's interpreted slides. It is desirable to have two or more Mohs surgeons in each unit.

ADVANTAGES AND COST-EFFECTIVENESS

Mohs micrographic surgery has a cure rate approaching 99% and 95% for primary and recurrent nonmelanomatous skin cancers respectively. Many systematic reviews of treatment modalities for primary BCCs have confirmed that tumours treated with Mohs surgery show the lowest recurrence rates compared with other treatment modalities [8]. Tierney et al. [2] also confirms the significant advantage MMS maintains reporting 5-year recurrence rates of 1% compared to standard surgical excision (10.1%), electrodessication and curettage (7.7%), radiation therapy (8.7%) and cryotherapy (7.5%).

Mohs micrographic surgery is a cost-effective procedure with treatment (including excision with appropriately clear margins as well as closure) often being completed within hours as opposed to days or weeks. Removing the least amount of nonneoplastic tissue, while maintaining adequate surgical margins allows for better functional preservation and cosmesis. As opposed to traditional surgical excision, 32–39% of these cases require a second procedure for clear margins leading to removal of greater tissue volumes which may have ramifications for both functional and aesthetic outcomes [2].

The average cost of Mohs micrographic surgery is $1263 (BCC cheek) and $1131 (SCC arm) [9]. According to a single centre randomised control trial completed in the Netherlands the total treatment costs of MMS are significantly higher in comparison to standard excision (cost difference: primary BCC, €254; 95% confidence interval, and recurrent BCC, €249; 95% confidence interval) [10]. The higher costs were mainly due to staff and theatre costs. The regression analysis showed that location and histopathologic sub-type had no effect on the cost-difference between the groups.

While the single advanced procedure is more costly than standard surgical excision, overall MMS is cost-effective as multiple surgeries are rarely subsequently required, the procedure is completed in a matter of hours and cure rates are extremely high.

Limitations

While Mohs surgery is highly effective in successfully treating a variety of skin cancers, often with multidisciplinary input, there are some limitations.

Patient factors, co-morbidities and tumour extent may be prohibitive. It may not be suitable for elderly patients who may be more suited to other treatment modalities such as radiotherapy.

Although a cutaneous malignancy clinically and histologically looks to be fully excised, if the tumour is noncontiguous or multifocal or contains satellite lesions (i.e. foci of tumour cells distant to the treated site) recurrence may occur. MMS is labour intensive and requires multiple team members and often multidisciplinary input. There are a limited number of MMS units and therefore access to this form of surgery may be restricted.

However, the benefits of this surgical technique often outweigh the risks and should be considered in all patients who would have otherwise been fit for standard surgical excision and who satisfy the MMS indications (see **Table 9.1**).

Key points for clinical practice

- Mohs micrographic surgery is a highly specialised form of surgery used to remove a variety of skin cancers, especially basal cell and squamous cell carcinomas.
- Skin cancers can be fully removed with maximum retention of normal tissue allowing for functional preservation and a better aesthetic outcome compared with standard surgical excision techniques.

- Instead of taking weeks for a definitive histological diagnosis assessing if tumour margins are clear with conventional surgical excision, removal of the tumour, closure of the defect and confirmation that it has been fully excised can be completed in a matter of hours with MMS.
- It is ideal for tumour sites such as the eyelids, lips, nose, ears and genitals, where tissue conservation is most critical.
- Skin cancer being most common malignancy worldwide, with incidence increasing on an annual basis, has and will continue to lead to an ever growing demand for Mohs micrographic surgery.

REFERENCES

1. Minton TJ. Contemporary Mohs surgery applications. Curr Opin Otolaryngol Head Neck Surg 2008; 16:376–380.
2. Tierney EP, Hanke CW. Cost effectiveness of Mohs micrographic surgery: Review of the literature. J Drugs Dermatol 2009; 8:914–922.
3. Shriner DL, McCoy K, Goldberg DJ, Wagner RF. Mohs micrographic surgery. J Amer Acad Dermatol 1998; 39:79–97.
4. Finley EM. The Principles of Mohs Micrographic Surgery for Cutaneous Neoplasia. Ochsner J 2003; 5:22–33.
5. Mohs FE. Chemosurgery: a microscopically controlled method of cancer excision. Arch Surg 1941; 42:279–295.
6. J Alcalay. The Value of Mohs Surgery for the Treatment of Nonmelanoma Skin Cancers. J Cutan Aesthet Surg 2012; 5:1–2.
7. British Association of Dermatologists working party report on setting standards for Mohs Micrographic Surgery services, recommendations of the British Society for Dermatological Surgery and British Association of Dermatologists, 2011.
8. Thissen MR, Neumann MH, Schouten LJ. A systematic review of treatment modalities for primary basal cell carcinomas. Arch Dermatol 1999; 135:1177–1183.
9. Rogers HW, Coldiron BM. A relative value unit-based cost comparison of treatment modalities for nonmelanoma skin cancer: effect of the loss of the Mohs multiple surgery reduction exemption. J Am Acad Dermatol 2009; 61:96–103.
10. Essers BA, Dirksen CD, Nieman FH, et al. Cost-effectiveness of Mohs micrographic surgery vs surgical excision for basal cell carcinoma of the face. Arch Dermatol 2006; 142:187–194.

Chapter 10

Vulval disease

Fiona Lewis

INTRODUCTION

The general topic of vulval disease encompasses several disorders including dermatoses, premalignant and malignant disease and vulval pain. This chapter will provide an update on key advances in the understanding and management of some of these. The recent changes in terminology of squamous vulval intraepithelial neoplasia (VIN) and vulval pain will also be discussed.

LICHEN SCLEROSUS

Lichen sclerosus (LS) is one of the most common dermatoses to affect the genital skin and if not diagnosed and managed early in its course, can lead to scarring and functional problems. It is well established that the first line treatment for LS is an ultrapotent topical steroid. However, this has largely been based on relatively small case series with only seven randomized controlled trials (RCTs) being included in the Cochrane review on the management of LS [1]. Evidence for the optimum regimen of treatment has been lacking, but recent papers have addressed some of the dilemmas associated with this.

Traditionally, a 3-month induction regimen reducing the frequency of application of 0.05% clobetasol propionate ointment has been used. After this period, treatment is then applied as needed for recurrent symptoms, or in those patients requiring more treatment to control their symptoms, this can be applied regularly once or twice a week. Previous studies have confirmed the efficacy of the potent topical steroid mometasone furoate 0.1% in the treatment of vulval LS. An RCT has now shown that this is equally effective as clobetasol propionate 0.05% ointment as an induction regimen [2]. The same group then confirmed that a tapering regimen using mometasone furoate 0.1% over 3 months is as effective as continuous treatment [3].

The role of both the topical calcineurin inhibitors tacrolimus and pimecrolimus in the treatment of LS has been reported in small studies. There have been some concerns about the possibility of potentiating malignancy and reactivating infection with these treatments. A randomized prospective study of 55 patients treated with either 0.05% clobetasol propionate or tacrolimus 0.1% showed that topical clobetasol propionate was significantly more effective in treating vulval LS based on the improvement in symptoms and clinical signs [4].

Fiona Lewis MD, FRCP St John's Institute of Dermatology, Guy's & St Thomas' NHS Trust, London, UK. Email: Fiona.Lewis@gsst.nhs.uk (for correspondence)

Most studies report results at the end of the study period and few have looked at the long-term management of LS. A recent prospective cohort study of 507 adult females with vulval LS looked at continuing treatment to achieve normal skin texture and colour and relief of symptoms [5]. A variety of topical steroid regimens individualised to the patient was shown to reduce the incidence of adhesions and scarring and also may influence the risk of malignant change as no patients who were compliant with treatment developed a squamous cell carcinoma (SSC) or VIN. A similar study in girls with pre-pubertal LS confirmed that maintenance treatment produced the best outcomes [6]. Thirty one of 33 patients (93.93%) who were adherent with treatment had complete remission with no progression or scarring. This contrasted with 69.23% of the non-adherent group who had disease progression and 23% developed further scarring.

EROSIVE LICHEN PLANUS

The most common form of lichen planus (LP) affecting the vulva is erosive LP. Although presenting in the genital area, it is increasingly recognised that erosive LP is a multi-site disease and it is important to exclude disease elsewhere, including the vagina, oesophagus, lacrimal ducts and external auditory meatus [7]. Treatment aims to improve symptoms and preserve function as the scarring can be significant.

A Delphi consensus exercise has suggested diagnostic criteria for erosive LP [8]. This has been confirmed in a case series of 72 patients [9]. The diagnostic criteria that are supportive of a diagnosis of erosive vulvo-vaginal LP are:
- Well demarcated erosions or erythema at the vaginal introitus
- Presence of hyperkeratotic border to the lesions or Wickham's striae
- Symptoms of pain and burning
- Scarring or loss of vulval architecture
- Presence of vaginal inflammation
- Involvement of other mucosal surfaces
- Presence of a well-defined inflammatory band involving the dermoepidermal junction
- Presence of a dermal lymphocytic infiltrate
- Signs of basal layer degeneration

The presence of at least three of these criteria is suggested to make the diagnosis. The histological diagnosis is not always easy in erosive LP and there are a subset of patients with clinical features of erosive LP where histology shows a regenerative vulvitis with loss of maturation and nuclear changes. It is very important to distinguish this from differentiated VIN [10].

There is little evidence for the most appropriate treatment in genital LP and management often needs to be prolonged and tailored to the individual patient. Ultra-potent topical steroids are generally used as first line treatment, and there is some evidence for the use of calcineurin inhibitors but they are poorly tolerated. There has been some recent interest in the use of photodynamic therapy (PDT) with an RCT showing a reduction in clinical scores similar in groups treated with genital PDT and topical corticosteroids [11]. The reduction in pain visual analogue scores were maintained at 24 weeks in those treated with PDT and less topical steroid was required by these patients after initial treatment. Anecdotal cases reports describe the use of rituximab in severe cases [12] but lichenoid reactions have been described as a side effect of biologic treatments so their use may be limited.

VULVAL CROHN'S DISEASE

Crohn's disease can involve the vulva with or without concomitant gastrointestinal disease. A clinical study of 22 patients and their response to treatment showed that 64% had gastrointestinal Crohn's disease co-existing with vulval disease [13]. Treatment remains challenging. In this study, topical steroids were found to be very useful. Azathioprine was helpful in 57% of patients. The anti-TNF agents infliximab and adalimumab were of benefit in 56% and 71% of patients respectively. Interestingly, those with vulval disease alone had a poorer clinical response than the group with vulval and gastrointestinal disease. The bowel involvement often responded well while the cutaneous genital disease remained active. The reasons for this remain unclear.

VULVAL INTRAEPITHELIAL NEOPLASIA

It is recognised that there are two pathways that are involved in the development of vulval squamous cancer. The 2003 classification of VIN included undifferentiated or usual type and differentiated VIN. Undifferentiated VIN is related to high-risk types (predominantly 16 and 18) of human papilloma virus (HPV). Differentiated VIN is not related to HPV infection, but can develop on a background of a chronic inflammatory skin disease such as LS. Undifferentiated VIN is the precursor of about 20% of vulval SCC but differentiated VIN is much more likely to develop invasive disease and leads to 80% of vulval SCC. It is often only diagnosed in the surrounding epithelium when an invasive SCC is excised.

Terminology

The Lower Anogenital Squamous Terminology (LAST) was introduced in 2012 [14] to unify the nomenclature of squamous lesions of the whole female lower genital tract. This uses the terms low-grade squamous intraepithelial lesion (LSIL) for HPV infections including external genital warts and high-grade intraepithelial lesion (HSIL) for premalignant disease, previously termed undifferentiated VIN. However, this classification raises two dilemmas with regard to vulval lesions. Firstly, as the term LSIL includes warts/condylomas, there is a risk that these are over-treated because they are included in this classification of pre-malignant disease. The previous term VIN 1 was abandoned as the basal changes seen are often reactive to inflammation or infection and surgical excision is unnecessary. They do not require treatment unless symptomatic. The second issue relates to differentiated VIN. This is a very important entity, having a high rate of progression to invasive malignancy. The International Society for the Study of Vulvo-vaginal Disease (ISSVD) has therefore proposed a modification to the LAST terminology (**Table 10.1**)

Table 10.1. ISSVD Classification of vulval intraepithelial neoplasia
LSIL – including flat condyloma or HPV effect
HSIL – previously termed usual or undifferentiated VIN
Differentiated VIN
Abbreviations: ISSVD, International Society for the Study of Vulvo-vaginal Disease; LSIL, low-grade squamous intraepithelial lesion; HSIL, high-grade intraepithelial lesion; HPV, human papilloma virus; VIN, vulval intraepithelial neoplasia.

emphasising that LSILs are due to HPV effect and may self-resolve [15], and including the entity of differentiated VIN. The WHO classification of vulval tumours has also been revised to include the differentiated form of VIN.

Management

The management of VIN can be surgical or medical. For small lesions that are easily excised, surgery is effective. However, as the aetiology relates to HPV, there is always a risk of recurrent disease. A Cochrane review of treatment included medical and surgical interventions [16]. This shows that there can be recurrence in up to 50% of patients after surgery. Randomised trials of topical imiquimod versus placebo show a complete response rate of 58% at 5–6 months versus 0% in the placebo group. One included trial of imiquimod versus topical cidofovir showed equivalent benefit so may be an alternative. However, longer follow-up studies are needed to see if the response is maintained. There are no trials comparing medical and surgical options and a combined approach is often required in these patients.

The HPV vaccine is known to reduce the rates of HPV related disease including HPV related VIN. In a population of women diagnosed with genital warts, vulval or vaginal intraepithelial neoplasia, a 35.2% reduction in the development of subsequent disease was seen after vaccination [17]. A new 9-valent vaccine (against HPV types 6, 11, 16, 18, 31, 33, 45, 52, and 58) prevented infection in disease related to the five additional HPV types covered and generated an antibody response that was of equal efficacy to the quadrivalent vaccine [18].

EXTRAMAMMARY PAGET'S DISEASE

The incidence of vulval Paget's disease is not known but in a large European study involving 16 countries, the vulva was involved in 83% of invasive extramammary disease [19]. The majority of patients have noninvasive disease and a recent review of the literature shows that the risk of progression into invasive Paget's disease or metastasis is very low [20]. Based on the evidence in the literature, a helpful protocol is suggested. Patients may be at increased risk of secondary malignancies and vigilance is recommended [21]. The site of the disease is important with perianal involvement being more related to colonic malignancy.

Treatment is unsatisfactory as there is a very high rate of recurrence after surgical excision. Further studies have confirmed the efficacy of topical imiquimod in noninvasive disease. A systematic review of studies which included 63 patients, 50.8% of whom had recurrent disease after surgery, showed a 73% complete response rate [22]. However, follow-up studies are needed to evaluate the long-term efficacy of topical imiquimod.

VULVAL PAIN

Vulval pain is a common reason for referral to vulval clinics but the diagnosis of vulvodynia still remains unrecognised by many health care professionals. The terminology with regard to the classification of vulval pain has evolved over many years, and has recently been updated further [23]. The symptom of vulval pain can either be due to a specific cause, or

Table 10.2: 2015 Consensus Terminology and Classification of Persistent Vulval Pain and Vulvodynia
Vulval pain caused by a specific disorder (Women may have both a specific disorder, e.g. LS and vulvodynia)
• Infectious • Inflammatory • Neoplastic • Neurologic • Trauma • Iatrogenic, e.g. postoperative, radiation • Hormonal deficiencies, e.g. genitourinary syndrome of menopause (previously termed vulvo-vaginal atrophy)
Vulvodynia – vulval pain of at least 3 months' duration, without clear identifiable cause, which may have potential associated factors
• Generalised or localised or mixed • Provoked or spontaneous or mixed • Onset – primary or secondary • Temporal pattern (intermittent, persistent, constant, immediate, delayed)

more commonly is seen in women without any obvious cause and is due to a neuropathic disorder. A range of disorders can lead to vulval pain and these have been expanded in the most recent terminology (**Table 10.2**). The diagnosis of vulvodynia should be used for vulval pain of at least 3 months duration where there is no clear identifiable cause. The aetiology of vulvodynia remains unclear but it is hypothesised that there may be a combination of factors that cause the problem and this may differ between individuals. Identifying these factors can be helpful in targeting treatment [24]. For example, pelvic floor hypertonicity can lead to chronic functional changes especially in women with localised provoked vulvodynia [25]. This group may therefore benefit more from physiotherapy than patients with generalised spontaneous vulvodynia.

Specific sub-types of vulvodynia are recognised with classic symptom complexes described by patients. The pain may be localised or generalised, and can be provoked (most typically by touch or pressure) or spontaneous. Some patients have an overlap or mixed picture. It has been known for some time that a group of patients with an inflammatory dermatosis such as LS or LP can also have vulvodynia, where the inflammation is well treated, but the patient continues to experience pain. This is included in the current classification. Other pain syndromes are seem more commonly in patients with vulvodynia with interstitial cystitis or painful bladder syndrome being most frequently associated [26].

The management of patients with vulvodynia requires an individualised and multidisciplinary approach, that must also take into account the psychosexual factors that can be involved in the condition.

CONCLUSION

The recent research in vulval disease has confirmed previous studies on some treatment modalities with more rigorous methodology. Updated classifications should help to stratify patients in future research studies and hence develop more appropriate treatments to specific disease variants.

Key points for clinical practice

- Studies have confirmed the efficacy of potent topical steroids for the treatment of vulval lichen sclerosus.
- The new classification for squamous VIN includes low and high grade virally induced lesion and also differentiated VIN associated with chronic inflammatory dermatoses.
- Vulvodynia may have different causative factors and associated co-morbidities.

REFERENCES

1. Chi CC, Kitschig G, Baldo M, Brackenbury F, Lewis F, Wojnarowska F. Topical interventions of genital lichen sclerosus (Review), Cochrane Database Syst Rev 2011; 12:CD008240.
2. Virgili A, Borghi A, Toni G, et al. First randomized trial on clobetasol propionate and mometasone furoate in the treatment of vulvar lichen sclerosus: results of efficacy and tolerability. Brit J Dermatol 2014; 171:388–396.
3. Borghi A, Corazza M, Minghetti S, et al. Continuous versus tapering application of the potent topical corticosteroid mometasone furoate in the treatment of vulvar lichen sclerosus: results from a randomized trial. Brit J Dermatol 2015; 173:1381–1386.
4. Funaro D, Lovett A, Leroux N, Powell J. A double-blind, randomized prospective study evaluating topical clobetasol propionate 0.05% versus topical tacrolimus 0.1% in patients with vulvar lichen sclerosus. J Am Acad Dermatol 2014; 71:84–91.
5. Lee A, Bradford J, Fischer G. Long-term management of adult vulvar lichen sclerosus. A prospective cohort study of 507 women. JAMA Dermatol 2015; 151:1061–1067.
6. Ellis E, Fischer G. Prepubertal-onset vulvar lichen sclerosus: the importance of maintenance therapy in long-term outcomes. Pediatr Dermatol 2015; 32:461–467.
7. Lewis FM, Bogliatto F. Erosive vulval lichen planus – a diagnosis not to be missed: a clinical review. Eur J Obstet Gynecol Reprod Biol 2013; 171:214–219.
8. Simpson RC, Thomas KS, Leighton P, Murphy R. Diagnostic criteria for erosive lichen planus affecting the vulva: an international electronic-Delphi consensus exercise. Brit j Dermatol 2013; 169:337–343.
9. Cheng H, Oakley A, Rowan D, Lamont D. Diagnostic criteria in 72 women with erosive vulvovaginal lichen planus. Australas J Dermatol 2015.
10. Day T, Bowden N, Jaciback K, et al. Distinguishing erosive lichen planus from differentiated vulvar intra-epithelial neoplasia. J Lower Gen Tract Dis 2016; 20:174–179.
11. Helgesen AL, Warloe T, Pripp AH, et al. Vulvo-vaginal photodynamic therapy versus topical corticosteroids in genital erosive lichen planus: a randomized controlled trial. BJD 2015; 173:1156–1162.
12. Heelan K, McAleer MA, Roche L, et al. Intractable erosive lichen planus treated successfully with rituximab. Brit J Dermatol 2015; 172:338–340.
13. Laftah Z, Bailey C, Zaheri S, et al. Vulval Crohn's disease: a clinical study of 22 patients. J Crohns Colitis 2015; 9:318–325.
14. Darragh TM, Colgan TJ, Thomas Coz J, et al. The Lower Anogenital Squamous Terminology project for HPV associated lesions: background and consensus recommendations from the College of American Pathologists and the American Society for Colposcopy and cervical pathology. Int J Gynecol Pathol 2013; 32:76–115.
15. Bornstein J, Goldstein A, Stockdale C, et al. 2015 ISSVD, ISSWSH and IPPS consensus terminology and classification of persistent vulvar pain and vulvodynia. J Lower Gen tract Dis 2016; 20:126–130.
16. Lawrie TA, Nordin A, Chakrabati M, et al. Medical and surgical interventions for the treatment of usual-type vulval intraepithelial neoplasia. Cochrane Database Syst Rev 2016:CD011837.
17. Joura EA, Garland SM, Paavonen J, et al. Effect of the human papilloma virus (HPV) quadrivalent vaccine in a subgroup of women with cervical and vulvar disease: retrospective pooled analysis of trial data. Brit Med J 2012; 344:e1401.
18. Joura EA, Guiliano AR, Ivensen OE, et al. A 9-valent HPV vaccine against infection and intraepithelial neoplasia in women. N Engl J Med 2015; 372:711–723.

19. Van der Zwan JM, Siesling S, et al. Invasive extramammary Paget's disease and the risk for secondary tumours in Europe. Eur J Surg Oncol 2012; 38:214–221.
20. Van der Linden M, Meeuwis KAP, Bulten J, et al. Paget disease of the vulva. Crit Rev Oncol Haematol 2016; 101:60–74.
21. Karam A, Dorigo O. Increased risk and pattern of secondary malignancies in patients with invasive extramammary Paget's disease. Brit J Dermatol 2014; 170:661–671.
22. Machida H, Moeini A, Roman LD, Matsuo K. Effects of imiquimod on vulvar Paget's disease: a systematic review of literature. Gynecol Oncol 2015;139:165-71.
23. Bornstein J, Bogliatto F, Haefner HK, et al. The 2015 ISSVD (International Society for the Study of Vulvo-vaginal Disease) terminology of vulvar squamous intra-epithelial lesions. Obstet Gynecol 2016; 127:264–268.
24. Falsetta ML, Foster DC, Bonham Ad, Phipps RP. A review of the available clinical therapies for vulvodynia management and new data implicating pro-inflammatory mediators in pain elicitation. BJOG 2017; 124:210–218.
25. Morin M, Bergeron S, Khalife S, et al. Morphometry of the pelvic floor muscles in women with and without provoked vestibulodynia using 4D ultrasound. J Sex Med 2014; 11:776–785.
26. Gardella B, Porru D, Nappi RE, et al. Interstitial cystitis is associated with vulvodynia and sexual dysfunction – a case controlled study. J Sex Med 2011; 8:1726–1734.